THE
Baby Boomer's
Guide to
NURSING
HOME CARE

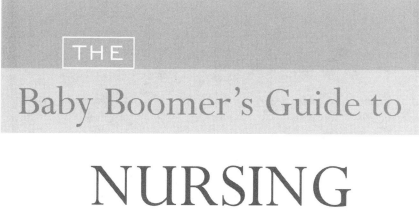

THE

Baby Boomer's Guide to

NURSING HOME CARE

**NATIONAL SENIOR CITIZENS LAW CENTER,
ERIC M. CARLSON,
and KATHARINE BAU HSIAO**

TAYLOR TRADE PUBLISHING
Lanham • New York • Boulder • Toronto • Oxford

Copyright © 2006 by National Senior Citizens Law Center
First Taylor Trade Publishing edition 2006

This Taylor Trade Publishing paperback edition of *The Baby Boomer's Guide to Nursing Home Care* is an original publication. It is published by arrangement with the author.

Published by Taylor Trade Publishing
An imprint of The Rowman & Littlefield Publishing Group, Inc.
4501 Forbes Boulevard, Suite 200, Lanham, Maryland 20706

Distributed by NATIONAL BOOK NETWORK

Library of Congress Cataloging-in-Publication Data

Carlson, Eric M., 1960–
    The baby boomer's guide to nursing home care / Eric M. Carlson and Katharine Bau Hsiao.
        p. cm.
    Includes bibliographical references and index.
    ISBN-13: 978-1-58979-323-1 (pbk. : alk. paper)
    ISBN-10: 1-58979-323-4 (pbk. : alk. paper)
    1. Nursing homes—Popular works. 2. Nursing home care—Popular works. 3. Baby boom generation—Nursing home care—Popular works. I. Hsiao, Katharine Bau, 1960– II. Title.
RA997.C32 2006
362.16—dc22   2005037658

∞™ The paper used in this publication meets the minimum requirements of American National Standard for Information Sciences—Permanence of Paper for Printed Library Materials, ANSI/NISO Z39.48-1992.

Manufactured in the United States of America.

Contents

Acknowledgments

HE AUTHORS and the National Senior Citizens Law Center thank the Harry and Jeanette Weinberg Foundation for supporting the writing of this guide.

Volunteer attorneys Jessica Soske and Georgia Burke contributed significantly to this guide. Helpful comments on initial drafts were provided by, among others, Stephanie Edelstein, of the American Bar Association's Commission on Law and Aging; Jody Spiegel, of the Nursing Home Advocacy Project at Bet Tzedek Legal Services; Alice Hedt, of the National Citizens' Coalition for Nursing Home Reform; Debi Lee, of the National Association of Local Long-Term Care Ombudsmen; Kristen Washburn, of Bay Area Legal Aid; Beverly Laubert, of the National Association of State Long-Term Care Ombudsman Programs; and Toby Edelman, of the Center for Medicare Advocacy. Their assistance is greatly appreciated.

This guide is based in part on the *Nursing Home Companion*, a California-focused guide written by author Eric Carlson while employed at Bet Tzedek Legal Services of Los Angeles. The National Senior Citizens Law Center thanks Bet Tzedek Legal Services for allowing this guide to incorporate portions of the *Nursing Home Companion*.

Portions of this guide's chapter 6, dealing with physical restraints and behavior-modifying modifications, are drawn from *20 Common*

Nursing Home Problems—and How to Resolve Them, published in 2005 by the National Senior Citizens Law Center.

Special thanks to the authors' families—Graciela Martinez and Diego Carlson; and Augustine, Alexander, and Elizabeth Hsiao Bau—for their patience during the many writing hours logged on evenings and weekends.

Introduction

O YOU KNOW anything about nursing homes? If your answer is *no* or *not much*, you are not alone. Most people typically know very little about nursing homes until an urgent need arises. Perhaps you or a family member will have a stroke or, due to Alzheimer's disease, will be no longer able to stay safely at home. All of a sudden, there will be much to learn and almost no time in which to learn it.

This guide explains the many laws protecting nursing home residents and gives practical advice on how residents and their families can obtain the best nursing home care possible. Here are some examples of the important protections discussed in this guide:

- A nursing home has an obligation to meet resident preferences (p. 107).
- A resident and the resident's family have a right to participate in preparing a written plan for the resident's care (pp. 112–14).
- Ownership of a home generally does not affect a resident's eligibility for Medicaid payment of nursing home expenses, as long as equity in the home does not exceed $500,000 (pp. 65–68).
- A Medicaid-eligible resident has a right to be readmitted to the nursing home following a hospital stay of any length (pp. 160–63).

- The spouse of a nursing home resident automatically is entitled to keep from $19,908 to $99,540 of the couple's savings, depending on the state, without affecting the resident's eligibility for Medicaid coverage of nursing home expenses (pp. 56–58).
- A nursing home cannot require a friend or family member to take on financial responsibility for a resident's nursing home care (pp. 78–83).

The federal Nursing Home Reform Law became effective in 1990. Nursing home quality of care has improved since that time, but much improvement still is needed. A well-informed resident or family member can assist a nursing home in taking legal responsibilities seriously—leading to greater dignity and improved care for residents.

About *The Baby Boomer's Guide to Nursing Home Care*

Although many guides to aging and long-term care exist, until now no consumer guide has provided a thorough discussion of the legal rights of nursing home residents and the legal responsibilities of nursing homes. Knowledge of these rights and responsibilities can enable and empower a resident (or her representative) to obtain the best possible nursing home care.

This guide is written in a straightforward question-and-answer format. It is intended for use by elders planning ahead, nursing home residents, and their family members and friends. It is also a worthwhile reference for nursing home operators, attorneys, social workers, and others with a personal or professional interest in nursing home care. For consumers, this guide is best used in conjunction with nursing home visits; interactions with local Long-Term Care Ombudsman programs; and, when needed, consultations with a knowledgeable attorney.

This guide includes the following chapters:

Chapter 1   Eldercare Options: Types of long-term care, including at-home care, assisted living facilities, and nursing homes

Chapter 2   Choosing a Nursing Home: Factors in choosing a nursing home

Chapter 3   Paying for Nursing Home Care: Medicare, Medicare HMOs, and Medicaid

Chapter 4   Admission Process: Illegal discrimination in admission and nursing home admission agreements

Chapter 5   Moving In: Transition and safeguarding resident property

Chapter 6   Quality of Care: Assessments, care plans, improving a resident's condition, meeting resident preferences, and no discrimination against Medicaid-eligible residents

Chapter 7   Residents' Health Care Decision Making: Powers of attorney for health care, health care directives, and the right to refuse treatment

Chapter 8   Staying in the Nursing Home: Eviction rules and residents' rights to hold a bed during a hospital stay or be readmitted to a different bed following a hospital stay

Chapter 9   How to Resolve Problems: Tips for resolving a problem yourself or obtaining help from a Long-Term Care Ombudsman program, state agency, or attorney

About the Authors

This guide has been prepared by attorneys Eric Carlson and Katharine Bau Hsiao of the National Senior Citizens Law Center

(NSCLC), a nonprofit law firm founded in 1972. NSCLC defends the interests of seniors through nationwide advocacy, education, and policy development. Among other things, NSCLC conducts trainings on nursing home law throughout the country and publishes *20 Common Nursing Home Problems—and How to Resolve Them*. NSCLC offices are located in Washington, D.C., and Los Angeles and Oakland, California. More information about NSCLC is available at www.nsclc.org.

NSCLC works with and provides training and information nationwide to attorneys who represent lower-income older persons, but NSCLC does not have the resources to provide direct counseling or legal representation for individuals. For advice regarding a specific matter, please contact an attorney or legal aid organization in your community.

Important Note

This guide is based on federal law and is intended for general use. This guide is not a substitute for the independent judgment and skills of an attorney or other professional. If you require legal or other expert advice, please consult a competent professional in your area to supplement and verify the information contained in this guide. Relevant laws can change from year to year, so be sure that you have the most recent edition of this guide.

Eldercare Options
Considerations in Choosing the Right Long-Term Care

- Introduction
- Remaining at Home
- Assisted Living
- Nursing Homes

Introduction

A nursing home is not the only game in town. This chapter discusses nursing homes along with two other long-term care options—staying at home (in some cases, a family member's home) and living in an assisted living facility.

It is impossible to say that one long-term care alternative is always better than another. This section discusses the options so that elders and their families can determine which is best in their particular circumstances.

Who decides when care is needed and what care to provide?

Preferably, the elder makes the decisions herself, with advice and assistance from family members and appropriate professionals. Decisions regarding long-term care can be anxiety provoking, and it will generally be important for the elder and the family to have the elder make or agree with the ultimate decision. Like anyone else, an elder will be more accepting of a decision made by her than one made for her.

Ideally, the elder and family will have discussed possible options well in advance of the time that long-term care is needed. If the possible need for long-term care is discussed early and often, elders and families are more likely to perform effectively when a potential problem arises.

An elder's decline raises difficult emotional issues. On the elder's part, she may find it difficult to admit need and to accept a loss of power and independence. Her family may also have difficulty accepting the elder's decline and, in addition, will likely struggle with feelings of guilt over the inability to meet all the elder's needs.

Also, a family may not be in agreement over what is to be done. It is not uncommon for family members (often adult children) to be at odds over the arrangements made for an elder's care.

For most elders, staying at home is a priority. Moving out of one's home can be a dreaded occurrence—both an admission of decreasing capacity and a loss of familiar and comforting routines.

To the extent possible, an elder should plan ahead and discuss with family members the point at which a move may have to happen. Consider what objective factors would indicate that a move should take place. Planning ahead will reduce the stress of decision making if and when the elder must consider moving. Communication among family members will help everyone involved feel confident that the best decision was made and followed.

A common reality, however, is that planning has not been done ahead of time. Furthermore, in many cases, the elder and the family do not even agree on the need for long-term care. Most commonly, the family is concerned about the elder's increasing frailty and forgetfulness while she insists that she's perfectly capable of taking care of herself.

This guide does not presume to instruct families on exactly how to resolve such differences of opinion—every family has its own personality and its own dynamics. In some families, confrontation is an everyday fact of life. Other families are less accustomed to conflict, particularly those involving difficult topics such as a parent's mental or physical decline.

This guide encourages families to tackle the tough topics head-on. If an elder is acting erratically or if the family is concerned about the elder's safety or the safety of others, the family should try to talk with the elder about those concerns. Avoiding the problem is ultimately no solution and will only lead to more problems in the future.

What happens if the elder is not capable of making decisions?

If an elder no longer has capacity to make medical decisions, the elder's family may need to ascertain whether advance planning has been done. See chapter 7 for more information on health care decision making.

Remaining at Home

What services can help an elder stay in his own home or a family member's home?

Various services available in many areas may enable an elder to stay in his own home or in the home of a family member, despite the elder's need for some assistance and health care. For example, in-home health care can be provided by a home health agency, through visits by a nurse or a home health aide. A personal care aide can provide assistance with dressing, cooking, chores, and other similar tasks.

During the day, the elder may be able to attend an adult day care center for meals, socializing, and services. Some adult day care centers are also qualified to provide limited health care. Adult day care centers may be particularly helpful for elders living with family members, if the family members work out of the home during the day.

Home-delivered meals are commonly provided through local senior centers and various charitable organizations. In many cases, these same organizations may be able to assist in modifying an elder's house to make it more accessible—for example, by adding grab bars in the bathroom or installing a ramp to the front door.

Actually, most at-home services are provided by family members and friends, whether the elder is living in his own home or in a family member's home. Of course, the feasibility of family assistance depends on whether the family lives in the same area and on the family members' other obligations at home and work.

The Medicare program may pay for home health care for Medicare beneficiaries who are considered "homebound"—that is, their mobility is so limited that they cannot be expected to leave the house for routine medical treatment. If the elder is terminally ill, the Medicare program can pay for hospice services, which are discussed on pages 120–21.

In many but not all states, the Medicaid program will pay for a package of in-home services for elders who are sick enough to otherwise be admitted to a nursing home. The idea behind the in-home care is that the elder benefits because he is able to stay at home, and the Medicaid program benefits because in-home care is less expensive than the nursing home care that would otherwise be required. Unfortunately, the availability of such in-home services is limited. State Medicaid programs generally have a cap on the number of Medicaid beneficiaries who can receive these in-home services during a given year, and many states have a waiting list.

What factors should a family consider in planning to care for an elder at home?

As always in these matters, advance planning is strongly recommended. Here are some issues to consider:

- With whom might the elder live, or how will she cope in her own home?
- If and how will the family share caregiving duties?
- How and for which services will family caregivers be reimbursed?

WORD TO THE WISE . . .

Be realistic. Family members may be motivated to do "whatever it takes" to keep the elder at home. Even with the best intentions, however, family members can only work so hard for so long.

Recognize that long-term care is more a marathon than a sprint. Plan ahead so that the primary caregiver is not driven to exhaustion. Ideally, family members and friends will share the workload. For example, one adult child could be the primary caregiver, and another could help with finances and medications. Out-of-town relatives might help with tasks that are manageable from afar and use vacation time to give the primary caregiver a respite.

Family stress and burnout can be reduced with planning. Regular check-in meetings among family members can also be valuable.

- What circumstances might indicate that at-home care is not workable—for example, caregiver burnout or a family's inability to move the elder from bed to wheelchair?
- How will a family caregiver get time off?
- Where will the elder move if the arrangement doesn't work out or needs to end for any reason?

Assisted Living

What is assisted living?

In general, an assisted living facility provides residents with room and board, assistance with activities of daily living (eating, dressing, toileting, bathing, etc.), and some level of assistance with health care needs. Assisted living is governed by state law, so the details of assisted living vary from state to state. In most states, an assisted living unit might be either a private unit or a shared room.

Most states use the term *assisted living*, although some states use other names to refer to this level of care. A state, for example, may use the term *personal care home* or *housing with services establishment*.

In the past, assisted living residents needed only minimal assistance with their activities of daily living, but this is changing. Increasingly, assisted living facilities are able to admit and retain residents who need daily health care or substantial assistance with activities of daily living. For example, some assisted living facilities can care for residents who are incontinent, have severe dementia, or are terminally ill.

Some assisted living facilities are small, with ten or fewer residents. In recent years, however, assisted living facilities are more likely to be larger institutions with one hundred or more residents.

Some assisted living facilities are affiliated with or adjacent to nursing homes (see following sections for more information on nursing homes and continuing care retirement communities). An elder may wish to consider the advantages of living in close proximity to a spouse who may need nursing home care.

To this point, most assisted living care is paid through residents' income and savings. In most but not all cases, Medicaid reimbursement is not available for assisted living care. In some cases, a state's Medicaid program will pay for assisted living services for those residents who are sick enough to otherwise be admitted to a nursing home. As explained in this chapter's discussion on in-home services, this type of Medicaid program is often subject to enrollment caps and waiting lists.

Further information about assisted living is available from the Assisted Living Consumer Alliance, at www.assistedlivingconsumers .org.

WORD TO THE WISE . . .

Consider the pros and cons of assisted living. It is both good and bad that assisted living facilities are now able to admit and retain residents with significant care needs. The good side is that elders have more options and that assisted living facilities may be more homelike than nursing homes. The potential bad side of assisted living is that, because assisted living facilities are much less regulated than nursing homes, the quality of assisted living can vary greatly. More often than not, an assisted living facility has neither a nurse nor a nurse aide on staff. An elder needing health care or significant assistance with activities of daily living should make sure that the assisted living facility is staffed and equipped to meet the elder's needs or that health care needs can be met by visiting nurse agencies.

What is a continuing care retirement community?

A continuing care retirement community offers all levels of care, from independent living to assisted living to nursing home care. Care is often provided in a campuslike setting with many buildings or houses, although some facilities consist of a single building. Continuing care is typically the most expensive option in long-term care. Oftentimes, a continuing care retirement community is affiliated with a religious denomination or other nonprofit group.

The benefit of continuing care is that an elder can move into a community and build ties while still independent and then move into appropriate levels of care as his needs for care and services change. For an elder who can afford it and is certain that a particular community is right for him, moving into a continuing care retirement community can be a long-term solution to many of the practical problems that can accompany aging.

Many continuing care retirement communities have long waiting lists, so an elder interested in continuing care should start shopping around sooner rather than later. Financial arrangements differ greatly from community to community. In a traditional model, an incoming resident pays virtually all his savings and income to the community in return for the community's promise

---

WORD TO THE WISE . . .

Carefully read any continuing care contract. Although continuing care retirement communities generally give the impression that an incoming resident is securing a home for the rest of his life, the contracts often give the community a great deal of discretion to terminate the contract and force the resident to move.

to care for him for life. Some communities require payment on a month-to-month basis, while other communities use a combination of these two models—the incoming resident pays a substantial initial payment, perhaps $100,000 or more, and also pays for care on a month-to-month basis.

Nursing Homes

What is a nursing home?

In addition to providing room and board, a nursing home offers assistance with activities of daily living, skilled nursing care, rehabilitation, medical services, protective supervision, and therapy. Other names for a nursing home include *nursing facility, nursing center, convalescent home, convalarium, long-term care facility,* or *sanitarium.*

Nursing homes serve people with great needs for assistance and care. Residents often cannot walk, and many need assistance with dressing, bathing, eating, and other activities of daily living. About half of nursing home residents have some form of dementia.

The staff of a nursing home includes registered nurses, licensed nurses, and nurse aides. Nursing homes must also have easy access to doctors and provide access to various health care services, including those of dentists and podiatrists.

Some nursing homes specifically provide care for residents with psychiatric disorders. Other nursing homes may offer specialized areas within the nursing home, such as an Alzheimer's disease unit. It should be noted, however, that all units of all nursing homes must be capable of providing care to residents with a psychiatric diagnosis or with Alzheimer's disease or another dementia. A nursing home's claim of specialization does not necessarily mean that the nursing home's care is any better than the care provided by any other nursing home.

Approximately 96 percent of nursing homes are certified to accept reimbursement from the Medicare or Medicaid programs. By accepting Medicare or Medicaid reimbursement, these nursing homes are obligated to follow the requirements set by the federal Nursing Home Reform Law. As discussed throughout this guide, the Nursing Home Reform Law establishes important protections for residents.

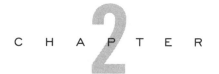

Choosing a Nursing Home

- Introduction
- Philosophy of Care
- Ability to Accept Payment from Medicare, Medicaid, or HMO
- Location
- Visiting to Determine Quality of Care
- Examining Inspection Reports
- Staffing
- Medical Care
- Referrals and Affiliations

Introduction

This chapter provides information on choosing a nursing home, including such topics as philosophy of care, location, visits to nursing homes, government reports, staffing, medical care, and referrals and affiliations. Payment and admission agreement issues are discussed in detail later in this guide, in chapters 3 and 4.

Unfortunately, the decision regarding the "right" nursing home is usually made when a prospective resident and his family are already in difficult times. Whenever possible, the prospective resident and his family should do preliminary planning. The best time to do this is before the need arises. A careful search of the best available nursing homes may prevent future disappointments and headaches. Inappropriate nursing homes can be weeded out, and the prospective resident can be familiar ahead of time with the most promising options.

What questions should be asked?

Choosing a nursing home may feel like buying a used car. The prospective resident or family member wants information but doesn't know what to ask and can't tell if the seller's answers are accurate. She may find herself asking a few basic questions, kicking the tires, and hoping for the best.

It's easy to get caught up in a nursing home's sales pitch—the talk about a home away from home, the remodeled dining room, the chandeliers, and so on. Prospective residents and family members are often insecure about the move to a nursing home, and as a result they may be overly inclined to believe a nursing home's claims.

This guide recommends that the prospective resident and family member think aggressively about what they want from a nursing home. They should ask the nursing home's staff members detailed questions about what the nursing home can specifically do for the prospective resident. For example, does the prospective resident want to walk around the block each day? Ask how the nursing home can meet that request. What if the prospective resident wants to wake up and eat breakfast on her own schedule each morning? Again, the question should be asked.

A nursing home's quality is more dependent on its employees and management than on its architecture or furniture. Pointed questions to the nursing home staff will quickly sort out if the nursing home is focused on resident needs. It is a good sign if the staff is willing to take steps to meet specific requests. On the other hand, if the staff is resistant to meeting requests or seems surprised or baffled by the idea of a resident making requests, then the prospective resident or family member may want to look elsewhere.

Philosophy of Care

What is resident-centered care, and how is this philosophy carried out?

For years, a principal criticism against nursing homes has been their tendency to treat residents as medical cases rather than human beings. Nursing homes have been trying to respond, and many now emphasize homelike environments and resident preferences. These nursing homes make decisions with an eye toward what is better for residents rather than to what is easier or cheaper for the nursing home.

This better way of providing care is commonly called *resident-centered care*, and many nursing homes have latched onto this term. Some of these nursing homes truly provide resident-centered care. But others don't. For some nursing homes, the adjective *resident-centered* may be nothing more than a marketing strategy.

Resident-centered nursing homes often participate in the Pioneer Network (www.pioneernetwork.net), the Eden Alternative (www.edenalt.com), or a similar program. A prospective resident or family member, however, cannot automatically assume that all participating nursing homes provide good care. It is not enough that the nursing home participates in one of these programs or, for example, has plants and pets. The staff should be able to explain what resident-centered care means—for the nursing home generally and the prospective resident specifically.

As discussed throughout this guide (see, for example, pages 128–29), a crucial issue is how and to what extent a nursing home truly will meet a resident's preferences. A prospective resident should mention three to five preferences and see how willing the nursing home is to meet them. For example, a prospective resident may want to eat frequent snacks or be taken around the block daily. A nursing home's response and expression of willingness to meet or accommodate specific preferences provide a strong signal as to whether the nursing home truly will operate in a resident-centered fashion.

Ability to Accept Payment from Medicare, Medicaid, or HMO

Is every nursing home able to accept payment from Medicare, Medicaid, and HMOs?

No. To accept payment from the Medicare or Medicaid programs, a nursing home must be certified to participate. As discussed on page 10, one requirement of certification is that the nursing home promise to comply with the federal Nursing Home Reform Law. A nursing home can choose to certify itself for Medicare only, Medicaid only, or both Medicare and Medicaid.

Even if a nursing home is Medicare certified, it may choose to certify only a percentage of its beds for Medicare reimbursement. Such "partial certification" may be allowed for Medicaid, depending on the state. Issues regarding partial Medicaid certification are discussed in detail on pages 152–53.

Most HMOs will pay for nursing home care only if the nursing home and the HMO have a contract.

WORD TO THE WISE . . .

Make sure that the nursing home can accept the type of payment that you intend to use. This is especially important if you are not Medicaid-eligible now but may become so in the future, after your savings have been spent down to Medicaid levels.

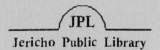

Jericho Public Library

#27   12-06-2011 3:47PM
Item(s) checked out to p100517912.

TITLE: The baby boomer's guide to nursin
BARCODE: 31325003545120
DUE DATE: 01-03-12

Jericho Public Library
516-935-6790

Thank You

Location

Which location is best?

If possible, the nursing home should be located near the prospective resident's family and friends, enabling easy access for visits. Isolation and loneliness are obvious and real problems for nursing home residents, and visits from family members and friends are high points in a resident's day or week. Residents with frequent visitors often fare better (emotionally and physically) than do residents without visitors.

If a prospective resident wishes to retain his doctor, he should find a nursing home relatively near to the doctor's office. However, the prospective resident or family member should first discuss the situation with the doctor. The doctor may be willing to visit only certain nursing homes, or the doctor may not visit any nursing home, no matter where it is located.

What type of neighborhood is best?

In general, the more peaceful, the better. A quiet residential neighborhood is usually preferable to a busy commercial strip, for obvious reasons. The environment in a nursing home can be chaotic enough without traffic noise and other neighborhood commotion.

Of course, there are exceptions to this general rule. Some prospective residents may in fact prefer a louder, urban neighborhood. A

WORD TO THE WISE . . .

Don't lose touch. Contact and rapport with people who live outside the nursing home can be important to residents. If a resident cannot live in a nursing home located near family members and friends, then a local church, synagogue, or senior center may be able to arrange friendly visits to the resident.

resident who loves urban living may feel trapped and isolated in a nursing home located in a sheltered neighborhood.

Also, some prospective residents may not have a choice of neighborhoods in choosing a nursing home. In the middle of New York City, finding a quiet neighborhood may be impossible. It will be similarly impossible to find an urban neighborhood in eastern Montana.

Some nursing home residents will want to get out of the nursing home during the day. For these residents, the neighborhood surrounding the nursing home is particularly important. A prospective resident and family should consider whether a neighborhood has sidewalks or is in other ways good for walking. A prospective resident and family also might consider whether a neighborhood has a park, senior center, shopping area, library, or other areas that the prospective resident may enjoy visiting.

In any case, prospective residents and their family members should not be overly impressed by the neighborhood in which a nursing home is located. Some excellent nursing homes are located in ugly neighborhoods. Likewise, some inadequate nursing homes can be found in attractive neighborhoods. Furthermore, many nursing home residents have physical or mental limitations that greatly restrict their ability to leave the nursing home for any significant period.

Visiting to Determine Quality of Care

What should a prospective nursing home resident look for during a visit to a facility?

The prospective resident and family members should visit each nursing home under consideration and then carefully look and listen. Are the residents up and dressed, or are they still wearing housecoats and robes in the afternoon? Do residents look well groomed?

Of particular importance, do staff members treat residents with respect? More specifically, does the staff have the time and inclination to stop and speak with residents? Do staff members appear to know the residents individually, or do they refer to residents by the residents' room numbers?

During mealtimes, residents should be given adequate assistance—it is a bad sign if trays are left in front of residents who cannot eat independently. In general, the atmosphere is better if residents eat together in the dining room rather than alone in their rooms. It should be noted, however, that a resident may choose to eat in her room rather than a dining room. A resident should have choice in the food served to her.

Appropriate activities should be provided. An activity schedule should demonstrate an effort by the nursing home to respond to residents' needs and preferences. Some residents may be capable of crafts or games and others better suited to simple exercises. Ideally, a nursing home should have some activities appropriate for those residents who retain significant mental and physical ability and other activities for those who have more limitations.

If the incoming resident is mentally alert, it is best if the nursing home has a significant number of residents who also are alert so that the resident more likely will have conversation companions. Understand, however, that turnover of residents is great in a nursing home and residents' conditions can decline so that the

---

WORD TO THE WISE . . .

Attitude is important. In a nursing home, so much depends on the staff members' attitudes. When visiting, observe as best you can how the staff relates to residents and how the staff members relate to each other.

character of a nursing home's population can change significantly over the span of just a few months.

Does the nursing home building itself matter?

The feel of the nursing home is important. Ideally, the facility should be homelike, attractive, and pleasant with adequate lighting and spaces for the various needs of the residents. There should be private spaces for visits or solitude and public rooms for socializing and activities. Sometimes activities have separate rooms, and sometimes the dining room and activity room are the same room.

Preferably, a safe space outdoors should be available. A garden area is a plus, particularly if interested residents can participate in the gardening.

Prospective residents and family members should not be overly impressed by chandeliers, ornate furnishings, or other touches of luxury. On one hand, a chandelier or an expensive furnishing may reflect a spare-no-expense attitude toward all aspects of the nursing home's operations. On the other hand, luxury touches may just be an attempt to divert attention from the nursing home's care and operation.

The traditional nursing home is like a hospital: long hallways with bedroom doors on each side. Some newer nursing homes break this mold. In one newer model, rooms are clustered around a living room area, like petals on a flower. The newer models are designed to increase residents' sense of community.

Do not assume that a nursing home has a sprinkler system for fire safety. Although national building standards require that recently constructed nursing homes be equipped with sprinkler systems, in many states an older nursing home is not required to have a sprinkler system. Fire safety is important—a fire in a nursing home can be catastrophic—so a prospective resident or family member should determine whether a sprinkler system is present.

What factors should be considered in viewing resident rooms?

Most resident rooms are shared. The prospective resident and family should consider whether a private room is wanted and affordable. Almost certainly, the state Medicaid program will not pay for a private room unless it is required for medical reasons.

When examining shared rooms, a prospective resident and family should check for size and privacy. Ideally, each resident will have some sense of privacy, particularly for visits and medical treatment. Private baths and showers are preferable, although showers in many nursing homes are provided in a separate shower room.

Call buttons should be easily accessible, and access to telephones and cable television is often desired. Of course, rooms should be wheelchair accessible and equipped with grab bars.

As discussed in detail on pages 93–94, a nursing home resident has the right to furnish his room.

What types of specialized equipment should be available?

The prospective resident and family members should look at rehabilitation rooms. Some therapies require particular specialized equipment.

WORD TO THE WISE . . .

Look behind claims of "special care." Some nursing homes advertise that they provide special care for dementia or other conditions. Such claims of special care may or may not be meaningful, because in most states there are no laws or industry standards for special care. Do not automatically accept claims of specialization: a nursing home's special care may be little more than a marketing strategy. If true specialization exists, the staff should be able to explain in detail what distinguishes the care from that of other nursing homes.

Some nursing homes specialize in particular services and have a good reputation for those services—for example, physical therapy or even ventilator care. Make sure the prospective resident's particular needs can be met.

To whom should prospective residents and family members speak?
In most nursing homes, a prospective resident or family member will be directed to the marketing director or admission coordinator. These employees, however, may have little knowledge of or control over the care provided by the nursing home. Of course, the prospective resident or family member should speak to the marketing director or other designated staff member but should also ask to speak to both the administrator and the director of nursing.

As discussed earlier in this chapter, the prospective resident or family member should ask staff members questions to see how willing they are to meet specific resident preferences. Good nursing homes adjust their policies to meet resident needs and preferences.

Beyond talking to staff, the prospective resident and family members should also talk to current residents and their visitors. The residents and visitors know better than anyone else the nursing home's pluses and minuses.

WORD TO THE WISE . . .

Don't be shy. Talk to residents and visitors. But don't have your conversations with nursing home staff hovering nearby. Ask staff members if you can be excused to speak privately with residents and visitors. If a staff member resists, you have an indication that the nursing home may not have a healthy attitude toward its residents.

A prospective resident or family member may wish to attend a meeting of a resident council or family council. These councils are discussed in detail on pages 167–69.

When should a prospective resident and family members visit?

If possible, the prospective resident and family members should visit the nursing home under consideration several times, at different hours and days—perhaps visiting on a weekday, during a weekend, and at night. They should make certain that residents' needs are being met during weekends and nights, when many nursing homes maintain a smaller staff. At least one visit should be done during a meal.

Examining Inspection Reports

What records are available for review?

Each nursing home that accepts Medicare or Medicaid payment is inspected approximately once per year. The most recent inspection reports are available from the nursing home; each nursing home must have the most recent report prominently posted and must make copies available upon request.

The inspection reports are also available from the state inspection agency. A state-by-state listing of state inspection agencies is included in appendix C of this guide, on pages 185–91. Summaries of inspection reports can be found online at the Nursing Home Compare website (see next section).

These individual nursing home inspection reports can be valuable in determining a nursing home's performance and its responsiveness to problems. While a nursing home rarely will have a perfect record, nursing home staff should be able to discuss any violation cited in an inspection report.

An important part of an inspection report is the nursing home's plan of correction. On the inspection report form, the violation is in the lefthand column, and the nursing home submits a plan of correction in the righthand column. Some plans of correction are thoughtful and appropriate. Other plans of correction are sloppy or, in the worst instances, outright hostile. If a nursing home submits a plan of correction that attacks the inspector or blames residents, the nursing home is probably not a pleasant place to live.

How is the Nursing Home Compare website used?

The Medicare program's Internet site (see p. 23) has a useful tool for assessing a nursing home. For every nursing home in the country that accepts payment from Medicare or Medicaid, the site lists quality measures, staffing levels, and inspection reports.

Quality measures are statistics on residents' conditions, taken from resident assessments. For example, one quality measure is the percentage of residents with a urinary tract infection.

Staffing

As mentioned, the prospective resident and family members should talk to various staff members at each nursing home under serious consideration. The administrator, director of nursing, and

---

WORD TO THE WISE . . .

Read the reports. It is helpful to read the inspection reports rather than to just rely on the online summaries in Nursing Home Compare. Not all violations are alike. It is not enough to know that a nursing home committed a quality-of-care violation. Did the nursing facility fail to document a particular treatment? Or did it fail to recognize or treat infected pressure sores? Unless you read the actual inspection report, you may not be able to tell if a nursing home's violation was trivial or significant.

USING NURSING HOME COMPARE . . .

1. Go to www.medicare.gov. Look under "Search Tools" and click on the link entitled "Compare Nursing Homes in Your Area."

2. Enter information about the nursing home for which you are looking, by state, county, zip code, or name of the nursing home. Click on "Next Step" or "Continue" until you reach a screen listing the nursing home.

3. Check the box next to each nursing home in which you are interested, and click on "Next Step" at the bottom of the screen.

4. For each nursing home for which you are interested, click on "View All Information about This Nursing Home." Various introductory data will be presented.

5. For detailed information, click on "Show All," near the bottom of the page. This will allow viewing of the following:

   Quality measures. Various quality measures, as reported by the nursing home (and not audited by any outside agencies), are reported here. Click on any measure and then on "Show All" to display the nursing home's quality measure information, along with state and national averages.

   Nursing home staffing. A chart presents the nursing home's staffing levels, plus state and national figures for comparison. Staffing levels are presented as staffing ratios—specifically, the number of staff hours divided by the number of residents.

   Inspection reports. A summary of the most recent inspection report is shown here, including all violations. Summaries of past inspection reports also are available by clicking on "View Previous Inspection Results," near the top of the table.

social services director may be helpful in discussing nursing home policy and practices.

During these discussions, the prospective resident and family members should be conscious of staff members' attitudes. Do the staff members seem to recognize the residents as individuals, and do they work to meet residents' individual needs and preferences? Or do the staff members routinely put all residents into the same schedule and activities? The following sections include issues that the prospective resident or family member may want to discuss.

Who is responsible for various tasks, and how does the nursing home ensure that those tasks are completed?

From a family member's point of view, the question is "Whom should I talk to if I have a complaint or a request?" Ideally, one or more staff members will be identified as the person or persons who will be responsible for certain aspects of a resident's care, and the nursing home will have a process to ensure that the necessary care is provided in the agreed-upon way.

How does the nursing home provide therapy?

Therapies include physical, speech, respiratory, and occupational therapy. (Occupational therapy assists residents in regaining or

---

WORD TO THE WISE . . .

Once the resident has been admitted, a family member will have to determine if promised care actually has been provided. This determination often requires reviewing the resident's medical records, which are available to the resident and resident's representative and by any other person who has been given permission by the resident or resident's representative. Access to records is discussed in detail on pages 108–9.

improving the ability to perform simple tasks.) Ideally, therapy services should be available seven days a week. Some nursing homes have therapists on staff; in other nursing homes, therapy services are provided by a visiting therapy service.

What is the ratio of staff members to residents?

Knowing staff levels—particularly those for the nurse aides who do the lion's share of the hands-on work—can be very helpful. Each day, a nursing home must post in a public place the number of nurses and nurse aides directly responsible for resident care for each shift. In addition, as discussed earlier, similar information on staffing levels is available from the Medicare program's Nursing Home Compare website (see pp. 22–23).

Do residents generally receive care from the same nurse aide?

The administrator or director of nursing should be able to explain how staff members are assigned. Preferably, nurse aides will be assigned so that each resident generally receives care from the same

---

STAFFING LEVELS

The Medicare program's Nursing Home Compare website expresses staffing levels in hours of resident care per day. Here is how staff-to-resident ratios translate to hours of care per day:

Staff-to-resident ratio	Hours of care per day
1 to 6	4 hours
1 to 8	3 hours
1 to 10	2 hours, 24 minutes
1 to 12	2 hours
1 to 16	1 hour, 30 minutes
1 to 24	1 hour

nurse aide. With regular assignments, the nurse aide is familiar with individual residents and accountable for their care.

Have staff members worked at the nursing home for a long time?

Staff turnover rates can be revealing. In general, lower turnover means that the nursing home more likely provides good care.

Among nursing homes in general, turnover rates are astoundingly high. Annual turnover rates for nurse aides frequently run at 100 percent or higher. In other words, a nursing home with twenty nurse aide positions might employ a total of forty aides during a year owing to the frequency of nurse aides quitting or being fired. Nurse turnover rates also are high—50 percent annually or higher.

An administrator or director of nursing may not be able or willing to cite staff turnover rates but should be able to answer some simple questions about how long employees have worked at the nursing home. A prospective resident or family member should ask which nurse aides have worked at the nursing home the longest and how long they have worked there. Or, more directly, the resident or family member should find out when the administrator or director of nursing started at the nursing home or how long the nursing home has been under the same ownership. Stability in management is a good sign.

Medical Care

What is the role of the medical director?

Under the Nursing Home Reform Law, each nursing home must have a medical director, who is a doctor that coordinates the nursing home's medical care. In practice, unfortunately, most medical directors have little or no involvement in the nursing home's day-to-day operations.

The prospective resident or family member should ask the nursing home staff about the medical director. It may be helpful to know the medical director's name and credentials, as well as his or her schedule and activities at the nursing home.

How and when are assessments and care plans done?

As discussed on pages 111–14, each resident must have an up-to-date assessment and care plan. A good nursing home will not just go through the motions, but will perform a careful assessment and then use that assessment to develop a care plan that combines medical expertise with the preferences of the resident and family.

The resident or family member should ask about the care-planning process. A staff member's answers may indicate whether the nursing home works with residents and family members to develop individualized care plans or, in a worst-case scenario, the nursing home sees the development of care plans as a worthless formality.

Referrals and Affiliations

Should a prospective resident use a referral service to find a nursing home?

A prospective resident or family member should not rely exclusively on a referral service. Some referral services may work solely from inadequate or outdated lists. Many receive money from nursing homes for each resident placed by the services. Referral services can be helpful but should be used with caution—they may have an incentive to place residents in particular nursing homes even though those nursing homes may not provide good care.

Can a prospective resident rely on a hospital discharge planner to find the best nursing home?

A hospital discharge planner may offer valuable information but is frequently under pressure from hospital management to move patients out as soon as possible. In too many cases, a discharge planner may refer patients simply for the hospital's convenience, hastily arranging for admission at whatever nursing home has an available bed. A resident or family member should not feel obligated to accept a discharge planner's recommendation.

How can I find someone who will give me an honest and informed opinion about particular nursing homes?

In many cases, personal connections are the answer. This is the time for the resident or family member to call up acquaintances who are doctors or nurses, who worked in hospitals or nursing homes, who lived in a nursing home, or who visited friends or family in a nursing home.

Social workers often have regular contact with nursing homes and can be quite savvy on the pros and cons of various nursing homes. Some social workers work in firms that specialize in geriatric care management; these firms, for a fee, will assist an individual or a family in setting up appropriate care, either at home or in a nursing home or some other long-term care facility.

On occasion, a Long-Term Care Ombudsman program (see pp. 172–73) will discuss particular nursing homes with a prospective resident or family member. Ombudsman programs differ widely in their willingness to have such discussions. Some programs consider such counseling part of their job, whereas other programs will provide little or no information.

Overall, finding someone with a knowledgeable and unbiased opinion is a hit-or-miss proposition. Such information is extremely helpful, but a resident or family member should be prepared to make a decision without such information, if necessary.

Should a prospective resident choose a nursing home affiliated with a religious denomination or cultural organization?

Some prospective residents may be more comfortable with a nursing home that has an affiliation with a particular religious denomination or cultural organization, or one that offers extensive bilingual services. The prospective resident's comfort level is an important consideration, particularly if he already has positive relationships with current residents of the nursing home.

It cannot be assumed, however, that a nursing home affiliated with a religious denomination is necessarily the best option. All prospective nursing homes deserve a careful evaluation following the factors set out in this chapter.

Even though affiliated with a particular religious denomination, a nursing home may well be open to individuals not associated with that denomination.

I've read this entire chapter, but I still feel uneasy. Am I missing something?

Not necessarily. Searching for a nursing home is not easy, particularly considering the emotions involved and the limited time that is usually available. Unfortunately, there is no scientific formula to determine the best nursing home. Although Internet sites provide an extraordinary amount of data about various nursing homes, that information is only a starting point for a search.

To the extent possible, set your sights high. Don't be embarrassed in the least about seeking competent personalized care. A nursing home generally receives $4,000 to $9,000 a month for the care of one resident. Given the significant cost of nursing home care, a nursing home's staff members should be willing to discuss how the nursing home can meet the particular needs and preferences of a resident or family member.

Paying for Nursing Home Care

- Introduction
- General Information
- Medicare
- Medicaid

Introduction

Nursing home care is expensive. Some nursing home residents have enough income or savings to pay privately for their care. The majority of nursing home residents, however, rely at least in part on the Medicaid program and, when available, on the Medicare program or private insurance policies. This chapter first will discuss general issues related to payment and then review Medicare and Medicaid.

General Information

How much does nursing home care cost?
Most nursing homes charge between $4,000 and $9,000 monthly for care. Rates sometimes differ significantly from state to state and

from region to region. Doctors' visits and special services may create additional charges.

Are insurance policies covering nursing home care a good investment?

There is no universal answer to this question. A full answer could require a separate book of this size and still would not give a yes or no recommendation.

A shorter answer is that each person considering long-term care insurance must examine proposed insurance policies carefully and give full consideration to his age, health, financial situation, and attitude toward Medicaid coverage. Consumers who are considering long-term care insurance should calculate what level of financial loss is unacceptable and should purchase insurance to prevent that loss.

In general, a person should not purchase long-term care insurance if he is eligible or soon will become eligible for Medicaid reimbursement. A policy should cover many types of long-term care—including home care and care in an assisted living facility or nursing home. Any policy chosen should contain a provision that will increase benefit levels if, as is likely, the costs of long-term care increase.

Long-term care insurance policies are governed almost exclusively by state laws, which vary greatly. Most policies will not provide coverage for preexisting conditions or mental illness (not including dementia), although sometimes state law forbids such limitations. State law frequently does not allow a long-term care policy to require prior hospitalization as a condition for coverage. Most states provide that a consumer may obtain a full refund within a short time after purchase.

Do any government programs help a nursing home resident pay for her care?

Yes. Both the Medicare and Medicaid programs pay for nursing home care under some circumstances, and the Veterans Administration covers care for a small percentage of veterans.

WORD TO THE WISE . . .

Premiums are not locked in. As a practical matter, long-term care insurance policies always allow the insurer to increase premiums. Don't buy a policy unless you can easily handle the premiums. Otherwise, a premium increase may price you right out of the policy, and you may lose the months or years of premiums that you have already paid.

Look for insurers with a proven track record. They are less likely to impose dramatic premium increases or go out of business.

Get some expert advice from a knowledgeable attorney or financial planner. Long-term care insurance is a sizable financial commitment.

Information about the pros and cons of particular policies is available from a state through its department of insurance or through state health insurance counseling programs. These counseling programs can be found by calling 1-800-MEDICARE or by visiting the Internet at www.medicare.gov/contacts/Static/SHIPs.asp?dest'NAV|Home.

The Medicare program pays only for short-term (one hundred days or less) nursing home stays and is subject to other limiting rules (as discussed later in this chapter). All told, Medicare payments amount to less than 10 percent of total nursing home revenue.

By contrast, the Medicaid program can pay for nursing home costs no matter how long nursing home care is needed. Medicaid payment constitutes approximately 60 percent of total nursing home revenue.

As discussed in this chapter, although many Medicaid laws are set by federal law, the rules for Medicaid can differ from state to state in significant ways.

WORD TO THE WISE . . .

Medicare is not a long-term solution. Prospective residents and their family members sometimes develop the mistaken notion that the Medicare program covers virtually all of a resident's health care needs. This definitely is not true for nursing home care. As mentioned, Medicare will at most pay only for a limited number of days at the beginning of a resident's nursing home stay.

What's the difference between Medicare and Medicaid?

Under both the Medicare and Medicaid programs, an adult beneficiary generally must be at least sixty-five years old or disabled. Under Medicare, a beneficiary or a beneficiary's spouse must usually have made certain contributions, through payroll deductions, to the Social Security program. A beneficiary's income and resources don't matter.

Under Medicaid, a beneficiary need not have contributed to the Social Security program but must have limited resources and income. Medicaid money comes from both state and federal governments, and some Medicaid rules vary from state to state.

In most cases, the Medicare program can be thought of as a health insurance policy purchased through premiums deducted from payroll checks. The Medicaid program, on the other hand, is a safety net medical program provided by the federal and state governments for persons who have little money to pay their medical bills.

Can a nursing home impose charges on top of the nursing home's daily rate?

Some nursing homes impose separate charges for various services or items (therapy sessions, catheter supplies, towels, etc.). These charges are improper in many circumstances, as discussed later in this chapter.

Private Pay If a resident is paying privately, the validity of a charge depends on whether the charge was authorized in the admission agreement. Specifically, a charge is invalid unless the resident in the admission agreement agreed to pay a specific extra amount for the particular service or item.

Even if a resident is paying privately and is obligated by the admission agreement to pay separately for certain items, he or his family may be able to save money by buying the items from outside the nursing home and then bringing them in.

Medicare or Medicaid Coverage If a resident's nursing home care is covered by the Medicare or Medicaid programs, a nursing home cannot bill separately for services or items covered by the program. As a practical matter, this means that the nursing home can charge any deductible or co-payment allowed under Medicare or Medicaid rules but can otherwise assess separate charges only for non–health care items or services, such as beauty shop services or television rental.

A nursing home's ability to assess separate charges under the Medicare or Medicaid program is limited because the coverage of both programs is broad. For example, the Medicaid program's basic daily rate covers payment for room and board (including laundry services) and all routine nursing services, therapy services, and over-the-counter drugs. The Medicaid program also covers a limited number of doctor's visits, plus prescriptions, eyeglasses, hearing aids, prosthetic devices, and ambulance trips. Although the Medicaid program does not cover beauty shop services, it does cover routine shampooing, hair cutting, and fingernail and toenail clipping under the daily rate.

Q & A: EXTRA CHARGES

Q. I just received last month's nursing home bill. My nursing home care is not covered by Medicare or Medicaid, so I pay privately. The nursing home is charging me $4,610: $4,000 for the monthly rate, plus $610 for other items and services. These "extra" charges include charges for therapy, catheter supplies, Kleenex, syringes, and bed pads. The nursing home's admission agreement did not list these extra charges. Do I have to pay them?
A. No. Because the extra charges were not listed in the admission agreement, you are not responsible for them. You should immediately request that the charges be removed from your bill.

Medicare

This section discusses Medicare generally, then reviews traditional Medicare, Medicare HMOs, and prescription drug coverage under Medicare Part D.

Who is eligible for Medicare?

Medicare is the federal program that is often the primary payer of the medical bills of people who are aged sixty-five and older, or disabled. In general, an individual is eligible for Medicare if she is at least sixty-five years old and she or her spouse has worked at least ten years in employment covered by Medicare. Because Social Security eligibility also requires ten years of covered employment, eligibility for Medicare is often tied to eligibility for Social Security. Specifically, if an individual is receiving Social Security retirement benefits, then she and her spouse are each eligible for Medicare, beginning on their respective sixty-fifth birthdays.

An individual may be eligible for Medicare before her sixty-fifth birthday if she is disabled. For example, an individual of any age becomes eligible for Medicare after she has received Social Security disability benefits for at least two years. Also, an individual whose kidneys fail becomes eligible for Medicare within three months, assuming that she or her spouse has an adequate work history. A similar rule applies to those suffering from ALS (Lou Gehrig's disease) but without any waiting period at all.

Even if an individual or her spouse does not have ten years of covered employment, she may become eligible for Medicare by paying premiums. If the individual is low-income and has limited resources, the state may pay the premium through a Medicare Savings Program or through Medicaid.

What's the difference between Medicare Part A and Medicare Part B?

Medicare Part A is commonly known as hospital insurance. Under certain conditions, Medicare Part A pays for a stay in a hospital or a nursing home or pays for certain expenses of home health care. In addition, Medicare Part A pays for certain expenses of hospice care provided to a terminally ill person.

Medicare Part B is commonly known as medical insurance. Medicare Part B pays for certain expenses of doctor services, therapies, tests, X rays, and medical equipment. Under some circumstances, Medicare Part B will pay for particular services provided in a nursing home or for home health care.

As discussed later in this chapter, Medicare Part C is the Medicare Advantage program that includes Medicare HMOs. Medicare Part D, also discussed later in this chapter, is the Medicare prescription drug coverage that began in January 2006.

WORD TO THE WISE . . .

Ask counselors questions. Every state has a state health insurance counseling program with volunteers trained to assist with questions related to Medicare, Medicare supplemental insurance policies, and Medicare HMOs. To get information on programs in your area, call 1-800-MEDICARE or visit the Internet at www.medicare.gov/contacts/Static/SHIPs.asp?dest'NAV|Home.

    As with any counseling program staffed primarily with volunteers, the quality of advice may vary, so be persistent in checking out the information that you receive.

At what point will Medicare pay for nursing home care?

Medicare Part A pays nursing home charges only for residents who need "skilled nursing or skilled rehabilitation services" on a daily or almost-daily basis. For example, "skilled nursing services," as defined by the Medicare program, include intravenous feeding, the treatment of widespread skin disorders, and the monitoring of residents who require relatively sophisticated evaluations. "Skilled rehabilitation services" include therapeutic exercises or activities, services provided by a speech pathologist, and occupational and speech therapy.

    Note that a resident may qualify for Medicare Part A payment of his nursing home charges if he requires only one skilled service. Note also that the skilled services mentioned here are examples only. The Medicare regulations clearly state that a variety of conditions may qualify a resident for Medicare Part A payment of nursing home charges.

    With respect to residents receiving therapy, nursing homes frequently—but incorrectly—say that Medicare Part A cannot pay unless a resident's condition is improving. Actually, prescribed therapy can justify Medicare Part A reimbursement even without current progress, if progress can be reasonably expected in the foreseeable future or if therapy is necessary to maintain a resident's condition.

Note, however, that most long-term residents of nursing homes are not receiving skilled services as defined by the Medicare program. The Medicare regulations say that routine personal care services—such as administering medications, maintaining catheters, and turning residents to prevent pressure sores—do not qualify a resident for Medicare Part A payment of nursing home charges.

WORD TO THE WISE . . .

Do not be misled by the term "skilled services." It is unfortunate that the Medicare program uses this confusing term, which leads many residents and family members to assume, wrongly, that all nursing home services are "skilled."

Who decides whether Medicare will pay the nursing home bill?

The nursing home makes the initial decision on whether a resident is medically qualified for Medicare Part A payment of nursing home charges. Consequently, a resident or family member should emphasize the resident's need for skilled services right from the start and should encourage the resident's doctor to do the same.

If at any time (including the time of admission) the nursing home decides that the resident is not qualified for Medicare Part A payment of nursing home charges, the nursing home must give the resident written notice of its decision. If the resident or family member believes that the resident is medically qualified for Medicare Part A payment of nursing home charges and thus disagrees with the nursing home's decision, he or she has the right to appeal the decision. The resident or family member begins the appeal by returning the written notice to the nursing home after checking a box that states,

> Option 1. YES. I want to receive these items or services. I understand that Medicare will not decide whether to pay unless I receive these items or services. I understand you will notify me when my claim is submitted and that you will not bill me for these items or services until Medicare makes its decision. If Medicare denies payment, I agree to be personally and fully responsible for payment. That is, I will pay personally, either out of pocket or through any other insurance that I have. I understand that I can appeal Medicare's decision.

While the Medicare program is considering the appeal, the nursing home cannot bill the resident for the nursing home charges in dispute. If the Medicare program eventually agrees with the nursing home and concludes that the resident was not qualified medically for Medicare Part A payment of nursing home charges, the resident or family member can appeal the Medicare program's decision through several additional steps. During these further appeals, however, the nursing home can bill the resident for the charges in dispute.

If a nursing home fails to provide a resident or the resident's family members with the required notice, the resident or family member can act on this error. He or she should request in writing that the nursing home submit a bill to Medicare Part A (even if the resident's medical condition may not meet the requirements described earlier in this chapter). Under Medicare law, a nursing home's failure to give the required notice may excuse the resident from paying the charges incurred during certain weeks or months, if the Medicare program finds that the resident could not have known during that time that Medicare Part A would not be covering the nursing home charges.

Q & A: MEDICARE PAYMENT FOR THERAPY

Q. My mother has been in a nursing home for about ten days, receiving physical therapy during the weekdays. The bills have been paid by Medicare Part A. I was told today that the therapy and the Medicare payment were ending immediately because my mother was no longer showing improvement and had "plateaued." I was also informed that my mother would be transferred down the hall because she could no longer be assigned a "Medicare bed." Is there anything that I can do? My mother is recovering from a stroke, and therapy is critical to her regaining her abilities.

A. Yes, there is something that you can do, because the nursing home's "plateauing" argument is wrong. Lack of improvement is not by itself a reason for discontinuing therapy or for stopping payment under Medicare Part A. Prescribed therapy can justify Medicare Part A reimbursement even without current progress, if progress can be reasonably expected in the foreseeable future or if therapy is necessary to maintain the resident's condition.

You should try to persuade the doctor and the therapists to continue therapy, and you should also file an appeal to force the nursing home to continue billing Medicare Part A for your mother's care. You will have two basic arguments in the appeal— that your mother has a medical need for continued therapy and that the nursing home failed to give proper notice of its decision to stop billing Medicare Part A for therapy services.

Finally, you and your mother should inform the nursing home that she is refusing the down-the-hall transfer. As discussed on pages 163–64, a resident has the right under the Nursing Home Reform Law to refuse any inside-the-facility transfer if the purpose of the transfer is to move the resident to or from a Medicare-certified room.

Under what conditions will Medicare Part A pay for nursing home care?

As discussed, Medicare Part A will pay for nursing home care only while a resident requires so-called skilled services. In addition, Medicare Part A may pay for nursing home care only if the resident enters or reenters a nursing home within thirty days after receiving at least three nights of hospitalization in an acute-care hospital. During the resident's first twenty days in the nursing home, Medicare Part A may pay all of his or her charges; during days twenty-one through one hundred of the resident's nursing home care, however, Medicare Part A requires that the resident pay $119 daily before Medicare Part A can pay the remainder of the nursing home charges. (This daily amount of $119 is effective for 2006 and will increase slightly on January 1 of following years.)

Medicare payment never continues indefinitely. The Medicare program will not pay for nursing home care for more than one hundred days per benefit period. A new benefit period starts when the resident has not received Medicare reimbursement for either a hospital stay or a nursing home stay within the previous sixty days.

As a result of these limitations, the Medicare program pays only a small percentage of nursing home charges. In summary, Medicare pays for nursing home care only if a resident needs skilled nursing or rehabilitative services. In addition, Medicare may pay 100 percent of nursing home charges for only the first twenty days of a resident's stay and only when that stay follows a hospitalization of at least three nights.

Will a Medi-Gap insurance policy increase a resident's nursing home benefits under Medicare Part A?

Probably, but in a relatively limited way.

A Medi-Gap policy (also known as a Medicare supplemental policy) is issued by a private insurer. Such a policy pays Medicare deductibles and co-payments but does not expand the services covered by Medicare Part A. Thus, in Medicare Part A coverage of nursing home care, the only possible benefit of a Medi-Gap insurance policy would be the payment of the $119 daily co-payment, if the resident qualifies for Medicare coverage for any day during days twenty-one through one hundred of the resident's nursing home stay.

To make comparison shopping easier, Medicare law has established twelve standardized Medi-Gap benefit packages, labeled A through L. Plans C through J cover the $119 daily co-payment for nursing home care, assuming that the resident qualifies for Part A coverage for the days in question. Plans K and L offer 50 percent and 75 percent coverage, respectively.

Is a "Medicare room" reserved exclusively for those residents whose nursing home care is covered by the Medicare program?

No. A Medicare room (or bed or "distinct part") is certified for Medicare Part A reimbursement. Medicare certification allows a nursing home to bill the Medicare program for certain stays in a Medicare room but does not prohibit a nursing home from using a Medicare room for residents who pay privately or through the Medicaid program (if the room also is Medicaid certified).

A resident has the right to refuse a transfer if the purpose of the transfer is to move him from a "Medicare bed." This rule applies whether the proposed transfer is to another room within the nursing home or to another nursing home entirely. This issue is discussed in detail on pages 163–64.

MEDICARE HMOS

What is a Medicare Advantage plan?

A Medicare beneficiary who is eligible for Medicare Parts A and B may instead choose to receive Medicare Part C from a Medicare Advantage plan. By enrolling in a Medicare Advantage plan, the beneficiary exchanges her regular Medicare benefits for the benefits promised by the Medicare Advantage plan. The Medicare Advantage plan must provide at least the level of benefits provided by traditional Medicare.

The Medicare Advantage plan comes in three forms:

- *Coordinated care plan*, which provides services through a network of health care providers. An HMO is the most common type. Other types of coordinated care plans include preferred provider plans, provider-sponsored organizations, and religious fraternal benefit societies.
- *Fee-for-service plan*, which pays health care providers for services provided.
- *Medical Savings Account plan* established by the Medicare beneficiary's contributions. Deductibles and co-payments for Parts A and B are taken from the plan until an annual deductible is met; then the plan covers 100 percent of Medicare-covered health care expenses.

The HMO (Health Maintenance Organization) is by far the most common type of Medicare Advantage plan. A Medicare HMO provides health care to Medicare beneficiaries who have signed over their Medicare benefits to the HMO. Once a beneficiary signs over his Medicare benefits, the Medicare program each month pays a certain set rate to the HMO, and the beneficiary receives all his Medicare-covered health care from the HMO.

What nursing home care is covered by a Medicare HMO?
By law, a Medicare HMO must provide a Medicare beneficiary with at least the services and items that Medicare would have provided for her. Therefore, a Medicare HMO must cover at least one hundred days of nursing home care for an enrollee who needs "skilled" nursing home care, as defined by Medicare law.

To attract enrollees, most Medicare HMOs eliminate the $119 daily co-payment for days twenty-one through one hundred of nursing home care. Some Medicare HMOs increase coverage to 150 days of skilled nursing home care per benefit period. In some instances this expanded coverage is a mirage, if a Medicare HMO refuses to authorize the promised nursing home care. Although on paper an enrollee may be entitled to 150 days of nursing home care, the HMO may stop payment after a few days, claiming that the resident no longer needs skilled nursing home care.

HMO coverage creates certain limitations. The enrollee is limited to the doctors, nursing homes, and other providers that either are employed or owned by the HMO or that have a contract with the HMO. HMOs generally have limited geographic service areas, which can make care access difficult for an enrollee who has traveled outside that area.

WORD TO THE WISE . . .

Think twice before signing your Medicare coverage over to a Medicare HMO. A Medicare HMO is not paid for each service provided; instead, it is paid a per-person amount monthly. The result is that a Medicare HMO generally has a financial incentive to limit the amount of care provided.

On the other hand, an HMO has a financial incentive to provide better care in order to keep an enrollee in good condition and reduce the need for future medical interventions.

Can a Medicare HMO force a resident to leave a nursing home?
No. A Medicare HMO makes decisions about the services for which it will pay. Those payment decisions do not give the HMO authority to force a resident to leave a nursing home.

Can a resident appeal a Medicare HMO's refusal to pay for nursing home care?

Yes, residents have the right to appeal. When a Medicare HMO terminates existing nursing home coverage, the HMO must give a written notice at least two days before the date of the proposed termination. If the Medicare HMO is denying coverage entirely, the notice must be given at the time of admission to the nursing home. The notice must be given to the resident or to the resident's representative.

The written notice must include the date that the coverage ends, along with the resident's right to appeal to a specified appeal agency under contract to the Medicare program. To appeal, the resident must submit an appeal request to the appeal agency by noon on the business day before the scheduled termination of coverage. In all situations, it is recommended that the resident make the appeal request as soon as possible.

The appeal agency is generally required to rule on a resident's appeal request within forty-eight hours. If the resident wins the appeal, the Medicare HMO will pay for nursing home care (but not necessarily for the HMO's maximum number of days). If the resident loses the appeal, he can appeal further but may be financially liable for nursing home care unless and until the appeal eventually is resolved in his favor. If the resident fails to pay, the nursing home may have grounds to evict the resident for nonpayment, as explained in chapter 8.

After signing her Medicare benefits over to a Medicare HMO, may an enrollee later switch back to Medicare benefits?

Yes, although some enrollees may have to wait. Long-term nursing home residents are allowed to leave a Medicare HMO effective at the beginning of the following month. Other Medicare HMO enrollees are subject to a lock-in that generally allows them to change or leave a Medicare HMO only once per year.

PRESCRIPTION DRUGS
Do Medicare prescription drug plans cover nursing home residents?
Yes. Medicare Part D offers prescription drug coverage provided through private insurance plans. This coverage is available to all Medicare beneficiaries, including those who live in nursing homes.

In general, Medicare drug coverage requires Medicare beneficiaries to pay an annual premium, deductible, and co-payments. If a Medicare beneficiary is also Medicaid-eligible, however, he will receive a Low-Income Subsidy (also called "Extra Help") toward payment of the premium. He will not be required to pay a deductible or co-payments.

A Low-Income Subsidy also is available to other low-income Medicare beneficiaries, including those on a Medicare Savings Program such as the Qualified Medicare Beneficiary program. The amount of the subsidy differs, depending on the resident's financial status.

If a Medicare beneficiary is entitled to a Low-Income Subsidy by virtue of being eligible for Medicaid, Supplemental Security

---

WORD TO THE WISE . . .

You may be eligible for Low-Income Subsidy. If you are Medicare- and Medicaid-eligible, you automatically are eligible for the Low-Income Subsidy. Even without Medicaid eligibility, low income and resources may qualify you.

More information is available from the Social Security Administration at www.ssa.gov/prescriptionhelp. Applications can be made at a Medicaid office or Social Security office. Individuals who apply at Medicaid offices will be screened for Medicare Savings Programs, which may enable them to receive additional benefits.

Income, and/or a Medicare Savings Program, then he will be enrolled automatically for the Low-Income Subsidy. Otherwise, a low-income Medicare beneficiary can receive a Low-Income Subsidy only by first making an application for the subsidy at a Medicaid office or Social Security office.

If a resident's nursing home stay is covered under Medicare Part A, prescription drugs are covered under Part A rather than a Part D plan. Coverage under Part A is discussed in detail on pages 38–42.

How can a nursing home resident choose a Medicare Part D plan?

The resident should examine the list of medications covered by a plan. For obvious reasons, she should choose a plan that covers the medications that she needs or is likely to need.

It is important that the resident (or resident's representative) take the necessary steps to sign up for a Part D plan. Choosing a plan is much better than being without Part D coverage or having a Part D plan randomly assigned (which will be done, after a delay of several months, for those Medicare beneficiaries who are Medicaid-eligible).

WORD TO THE WISE . . .

Nursing homes must ensure that residents receive prescribed medication. Even if a prescribed medication is not covered by a resident's Part D plan, the nursing home has an obligation to ensure that the resident receives the medication. If the resident is eligible for Medicaid, the nursing home must provide the medication under the regular Medicaid rate, assuming that no other source of payment is available.

How can a resident change from one Part D plan to another?

A nursing home resident can change his Medicare Part D plan once per month and once within the two months after leaving the nursing home.

Note that a Medicare Part D plan must provide a transition-period supply of medication for those who move from one care setting to another—from a nursing home to a hospital, for example— or for nursing home residents who change from one Part D plan to another. The transition-period medication must be enough to last for at least ninety days.

Medicaid

This section first discusses Medicaid for unmarried residents; it then reviews Medicaid for married residents. It goes on to discuss the Medicaid resource rules for all Medicaid recipients, concluding with a discussion of a Medicaid program's ability to recover its expenses from the estate of a deceased Medicaid beneficiary.

MEDICAID FOR UNMARRIED RESIDENTS

When will Medicaid pay for an unmarried resident's nursing home care?

An unmarried person is eligible for Medicaid benefits if he is at least sixty-five years old or disabled and his available resources do not exceed the state's resident resource allowance. In most states, the resident resource allowance is $2,000, and in virtually all other states the resident resource allowance is between $1,000 and $4,000. (A state-by-state listing of resident resource allowances can be found in appendix A.)

Availability of resources is discussed in detail on pages 64–69. It is important to note that a home is generally not considered an available resource as long as the resident's Medicaid application indicates that the resident intends to return to the home, and the resident's equity in the home does not exceed $500,000. As a result, possession of a home generally does not prevent or limit an individual's eligibility for Medicaid payment of nursing home care.

In contrast to the Medicare program, the Medicaid program is a safety-net program that does not require that a resident receive skilled nursing or rehabilitative services to be eligible for nursing home care. The key for Medicaid eligibility is that the resident needs nursing home care. State Medicaid programs set their own standards for determining when a resident needs nursing home care.

Does income matter in determining Medicaid eligibility?

A resident's income often is not relevant in determining whether she is eligible for Medicaid payment of her nursing home expenses. Income is relevant only after the resident has been found eligible, when the Medicaid program determines how much of her monthly income (if any) she will be required to pay as a monthly patient pay amount toward her nursing home care. The calculation of a monthly Medicaid patient pay amount is discussed later in this chapter, on pages 51–54.

In a minority of states, however, income is relevant for determining eligibility. In these states, Medicaid eligibility is denied if the monthly income of an unmarried resident exceeds a certain "income cap." The income cap for 2006 is $1,809 and will increase slightly in later years.

A Medicaid income cap leaves some residents in a predicament. If, for example, a resident has $1,810 in available income ($1 over the income cap), she is ineligible for Medicaid coverage of her nursing home expenses but unable to pay privately for the care. To protect residents against such a harsh result, federal Medicaid law allows over-income residents to place their "extra" available income in a trust. The resident has access to the money in the trust while she is alive, but after her death the remaining money in the trust is paid to the state.

These trusts commonly are called *Miller trusts*. Residents who might benefit from such a trust should contact a knowledgeable elder-law attorney.

Is a Medicaid-eligible resident required to pay any of his monthly income to the nursing home?

Yes, almost always, if the resident is unmarried. An unmarried nursing home resident is allowed to keep only a small amount of his monthly income as a personal needs allowance. The amount of a personal needs allowance varies from state to state, from a low of $30.00 to a high of $90.45 (in 2006). A state-by-state listing of personal needs allowances is provided in appendix A.

The rest of the resident's income—excluding the personal needs allowance—must be paid as a monthly health care deductible (frequently called a *patient pay amount* or *share of cost*). The patient pay amount is typically paid to the nursing home for the current month's bill but may under some circumstances be paid toward past months' nursing home charges (if the resident was not Medicaid-eligible in the month or months in which charges were incurred) or certain current and past medical bills.

Once the patient pay amount is paid, the Medicaid program then will pay any remaining nursing home charges for that month.

Q & A: MEDICAID COVERAGE

Q. I am single, have $1,100 in a checking account, and receive $900 in Social Security each month. In my state, the resident resource allowance is $2,000, and the personal needs allowance is $40. Will Medicaid help pay my nursing home expenses?

A. Yes. You are eligible for Medicaid because you have less than $2,000 in resources. You will be allowed to keep $40 of your income each month. You will have to pay the rest of your income, $860 monthly, to the nursing home as a patient pay amount.

How can a resident use the patient pay amount to obtain additional services?

The key fact is that a patient pay amount can be used to pay for health care expenses that would otherwise not be covered by Medicaid. As a result, a resident is better off spending her patient pay amount on a noncovered service than on a covered service. Once the patient pay amount is spent, the Medicaid program will pay for all Medicaid-covered services anyway.

Of course, for this strategy to be effective, the resident must have a relatively significant patient pay amount. Assume, for example, that the resident is obligated to pay a monthly patient pay amount of $500. If she pays the $500 for her current month's nursing home bill, the Medicaid program will simply pay the remainder of the current month's nursing home bill. But what if she pays the $500 on therapy, for example, that otherwise would not be Medicaid-covered? She receives therapy that she otherwise might not receive, and the Medicaid program pays all of the month's nursing home bill.

How can a resident use the Medicaid patient pay amount to pay for past-due health care expenses?

As explained, a patient pay amount can be used to pay for a service that would otherwise not be covered by Medicaid. A past-due health care bill qualifies as a noncovered health care expense under this rule, unless the past-due bill is the result of a failure to pay previous patient pay amounts. Thus, a patient pay amount can be used to pay for a past-due health care bill.

Here's a typical example. Assume that a nursing home resident is paying privately until his savings are spent down to $2,500. At that point, he cannot pay the monthly nursing home bill of $5,000, so he files a Medicaid application. Three months later, the Medicaid office denies his application because his savings exceed the resident resource allowance of $2,000. (He should have made a partial payment to the nursing home or purchased some additional item or service to push his savings below the $2,000 level.)

The resident then spends his savings below $2,000 and obtains Medicaid eligibility, with a monthly patient pay amount of $1,000. The nursing home bills the resident for $15,000 for the three unpaid months.

To pay off the past-due bill, the resident can have his $1,000 monthly patient pay amount applied to the past-due bill. Each month, the past-due bill will be reduced by $1,000, and the Medicaid program will pay all of the current month's bill. In fifteen months (at $1,000 per month), the past-due bill of $15,000 will be paid off in full.

A MEDICAID APPLICATION TIP

Applications can be retroactive. Federal Medicaid law allows eligibility to be granted for up to three months before the month of application. Note, however, that retroactive eligibility can be granted only if the applicant met eligibility standards for the month or months in question.

Can a resident retain additional income to keep up a home or an apartment while she is in the nursing home?

Yes, but only in some states and only if the resident's doctor certifies that she is likely to need nursing home care for no more than six months. Even under those circumstances, the "extra" income allocation generally is quite small—likely in the range of only $200 per month. Needless to say, this amount is rarely enough to maintain a home or cover a rent payment.

In general, unmarried Medicaid-eligible residents should not expect to have enough money to pay for maintenance of a home or apartment. Unfortunately, however, many residents have unrealistic expectations of retaining a home or apartment. Unmarried Medicaid-eligible residents often get themselves in financial trouble by maintaining a home or apartment with income that, under Medicaid rules, should be paid to the nursing home (or other health care provider) as the patient pay amount.

The basic problem is that the Medicaid personal needs allowance is not nearly enough to cover the costs of maintaining a home or paying rent on an apartment. Specifically, as shown in the state-by-state listing in appendix A, the personal needs allowance generally is in the range of $30.00 to $60.00 monthly. The personal needs allowance is small because it is calculated based on the premise that the resident's needs for room, board, and care are being met by the nursing home and that the resident needs only enough money to buy the occasional item of clothing.

WORD TO THE WISE . . .

Maintain a resident's home by renting it out. One way to maintain a resident's home is to rent it out. Assume that the cost of maintaining an unmarried resident's home is $400 monthly. If the home is rented out for $900 monthly, the resident can pay for the maintenance and still clear $500 monthly ($900 − $400 = $500). The home can thus be maintained, although the resident will ultimately not profit from the rental—the $500 profit from the home rental will be canceled out by a $500 increase in the patient pay amount.

The key to this strategy is that the Medicaid program considers the resident's net rental income, not his gross rental income.

A resident has no income and no savings. Will Medicaid pay for her clothing?

No, Medicaid only pays for health care expenses. However, if a resident has no income or almost no income, she may be eligible for Supplemental Security Income (SSI), a federal program that supplements a nursing home resident's income up to a total of at least $30 per month. The SSI program guarantees a certain income for persons who are at least sixty-five years old or disabled and who have limited income and resources. SSI is administered by the

WORD TO THE WISE . . .

SSI is not used often in nursing homes. Most residents already have income that exceeds the SSI payment amount, so they are not eligible for SSI. In fact, individuals often lose SSI eligibility when moving into a nursing home. This occurs because SSI payment rates are much higher when an individual lives in a house, apartment, or assisted living facility rather than in a nursing home.

Assume some typical facts. An unmarried individual is potentially eligible for SSI because she is over sixty-five years old and has less than $2,000 in available resources. She receives $400 monthly from a pension. In her state, the SSI standard monthly payment rate is $600 but is reduced to $45 for nursing home residents.

When the individual is living in her home, SSI will pay her an extra $200 monthly to supplement her income to the SSI level of $600 monthly. If, however, she moves into a nursing home, her SSI eligibility will end because her pension income of $400 is already higher than the SSI level of $45.

The bottom line? SSI payment is relevant for only those nursing home residents who have no income or almost no income.

Social Security Administration. SSI-eligible residents receive Medicaid without paying a patient pay amount.

The exact amount of a resident's monthly SSI payment varies from state to state. It must be at least $30 and rarely is more than $50. Applications for SSI can be made by calling 1-800-772-1213.

MEDICAID FOR MARRIED RESIDENTS
When will Medicaid pay for a married resident's nursing home care?

As described, the Medicaid program generally does not pay for nursing home care until a nursing home resident has spent down virtually all of his or her available resources—usually down to the vicinity of $2,000, depending on the state. As a result, before the 1990s, the spouse of a married nursing home resident was forced to spend virtually all of the couple's resources for nursing home care. This put the at-home spouse in a very difficult financial situation.

In response, federal Medicaid law was changed to allow a resident's spouse to retain additional resources, assuming that the spouse does not also live in a nursing home. The basic rule today is that an at-home spouse is entitled to one-half of the couple's combined available resources at the time the resident entered the nursing home, up to a maximum of $99,540 (for 2006).

Because basing a resource allowance on one-half of total available resources may be harsh for those couples with relatively limited resources, federal Medicaid law offers an alternative. Rather than retaining one-half of the couple's total available resources, the at-home spouse can instead choose to keep resources up to an at-home spouse resource allowance, set by the state. Under federal law, a state Medicaid program in 2006 must have an at-home spouse resource allowance of at least $19,908 but no more than $99,540.

A state-by-state listing of the at-home spouse resource allowance for 2006 can be found in appendix A. The listed amounts will likely increase in following years.

Remember, a home is generally not counted in calculation of available resources. See pages 65–68.

If a state has set its at-home spouse resource allowance at the highest possible level—$99,540 for 2006—there is no need to calculate one-half of the couple's resources. Because the "one-half method" is capped at $99,540, it never will be a preferable option in a state in which the at-home spouse resource allowance already is set at $99,540. This rule—that the one-half method is not relevant in a state that sets the at-home resource allowance at the highest possible level—will continue to be true in 2007 and afterward, because by law the cap applied in the one-half method is always identical to the maximum at-home spouse resource allowance.

Medicaid law provides a final alternative that is designed for couples who need to retain additional resources to generate an adequate monthly income for the at-home spouse. That alternative

WORD TO THE WISE . . .

Are the couple's resources more than double the state's at-home spouse resource allowance? If the couple's available resources (not including the couple's home) are more than double the state's at-home spouse resource allowance, the couple will be better off basing eligibility calculations on one-half of the couple's available resources. On the other hand, if the couple's available resources are less than double the at-home spouse resource allowance, the couple will do better by using the at-home spouse resource allowance.

As discussed, the one-half method is not useful in a state that has set its at-home spouse resource allowance at the highest possible level—$99,540 for 2006.

requires an order from a court or an administrative law judge and is discussed on pages 62–63.

In summary, the at-home spouse can keep whichever is greater:

- one-half of the couple's resources, up to $99,540;
- an at-home spouse resource allowance set by the state, which in 2006 is at least $19,908 but no more than $99,540, depending on the state; or
- an amount set by a court or administrative law judge, based on the amount of resources needed to generate an adequate monthly income for the at-home spouse.

Can a married resident become eligible for Medicaid more quickly by putting resources into the name of the at-home spouse?

No, moving resources from one spouse to the other does not affect eligibility. As discussed, in determining the Medicaid eligibility of a married nursing home resident, the Medicaid program considers the combined available resources of the resident and the resident's at-home spouse.

Is a married resident required to pay any of his monthly income to the nursing home?

Possibly. The resident may be required to pay a monthly patient pay amount, depending on the calculations explained in the following paragraphs. As discussed (see pp. 52–53), a patient pay amount is generally paid to the nursing home for the current month's care but may also be used for past months' care (if the resident was not Medicaid-eligible during the month or months in question) and for certain current and past health care expenses.

If a patient pay amount is required, it is taken from the resident's income, not the at-home spouse's income. Medicaid follows what is commonly called the *name-on-the-check rule*, which is as follows: if a check comes only in the name of the at-home spouse,

RESOURCES: MR. AND MRS. JACKSON

1. When Mr. Jackson entered a nursing home, the couple had $220,000 in available resources. Mrs. Jackson lives in the couple's home, which has a market value of $300,000. The state's resource allowances are $2,000 for residents and $60,000 for at-home spouses.

   The value of the home won't matter. As is discussed on pages 65–68, a home with equity of $500,000 or less is considered an unavailable resource if the resident intends to return to the home or the resident's spouse lives in the home.

   One-half of the Jacksons' available resources comes to $110,000, but this is reduced to the federal maximum of $99,540. Thus, the couple can keep a total of $101,540 in available resources—$99,540 for Mrs. Jackson and $2,000 (the resident resource allowance) for Mr. Jackson. In general, Mr. Jackson will not be eligible for Medicaid reimbursement until the couple's available resources are spent down to a total of $101,540.

2. Now assume that the Jacksons had only $150,000 in available resources when Mr. Jackson entered the nursing home. Again, Mr. Jackson will be able to keep $2,000, but this time Mrs. Jackson will be allowed to keep only $75,000, which is one-half of $150,000. Together, the couple will be allowed to keep $77,000 in available resources.

3. If the Jacksons had $100,000 in available resources when Mr. Jackson entered the nursing home, the couple will be allowed to keep a total of $62,000. The state allows an at-home resource allowance of up to $60,000, even if that amount is more than one-half of the couple's total available resources. The additional $2,000 is the resident's resource allowance for Mr. Jackson.

none of that income will be required to be paid as part of the resident's patient pay amount.

Nonetheless, an at-home spouse's income can matter because it can affect the at-home spouse's right to use the resident's income. The more of a resident's income needed by an at-home spouse, the less of the resident's income that must be paid as a patient pay amount.

From the resident's available income, the resident is entitled to a personal needs allowance, and the resident's at-home spouse may be entitled to a separate income allowance, as discussed in the following section. Whatever is left of the resident's income is paid as the patient pay amount.

How much of a resident's income can be retained by the at-home spouse?

Under certain conditions, the at-home spouse can take for herself some or all of the resident's otherwise-available monthly income. The total income taken by the at-home spouse—the at-home spouse's income plus some or all of the resident's income—cannot exceed a monthly income allowance set by the state within federal limits. For 2006, a state must set an income allowance of at least $1,603.75 but no more than $2,488.50. The lower limit will increase slightly on July 1, 2006. Both the lower and upper limits will be increased in 2007 and in each following year.

A state-by-state listing of at-home spouse income allowances for 2006 is provided in appendix A of this guide. In general, these income allowances slightly increase from year to year, depending on the state.

If an at-home spouse's housing expenses are relatively high, she may be able to retain extra income but only up to a total income allowance of $2,488.50 (in 2006). The extra income allocation consists of the amount by which the at-home spouse's housing costs exceed $481.13 monthly ($553.50 in Hawaii; $601.13 in Alaska; all figures apply to 2006 and will increase slightly in following years).

INCOME: MR. AND MRS. JACKSON

1. Mr. Jackson, a nursing home resident, has an income of $1,600 monthly; his wife has an income of $1,000 monthly. Mrs. Jackson's monthly housing costs total $1,081.13. The state's at-home spouse income allowance is $2,000, and its personal needs allowance is $40.

   Mrs. Jackson's housing costs exceed the standard amount by $600 ($1,081.13 – $481.13 = $600). Adding the excess housing costs of $600 to the at-home spouse income allowance of $2,000 produces a total of $2,600, but this is reduced to the federal maximum of $2,488.50.

   Thus, Mrs. Jackson is entitled to retain a total monthly income of $2,488.50—all of her $1,000 monthly income, plus $1,488.50 from her husband's income. Mr. Jackson is entitled to his personal needs allowance of $40, and Mr. Jackson's monthly patient pay amount is $71.50—his income of $1,600 minus his personal needs allowance of $40 and minus $1,488.50 that is allocated to his wife.

2. Now increase Mrs. Jackson's monthly income to $3,000, but keep all other facts the same. She is allowed to retain all of her income under the name-on-the-check rule but is not entitled to any allocation from her husband, because her $3,000 is already "enough" based on the Medicaid rules discussed earlier. Mr. Jackson now can keep only his $40 personal needs allowance. His monthly patient pay amount is $1,560—his $1,600 income minus his $40 personal needs allowance.

Housing costs include mortgage payments, rent, utilities, taxes, insurance, and condominium fees.

Note that housing costs don't matter in those states that have set their at-home spouse income allowance at the highest level—$2,488.50 in 2006—because excess housing costs can increase an income allowance only up to $2,488.50. Every year, the maximum state at-home spouse income allowance is identical to the cap that applies to the combination of an at-home spouse income allowance with "excess" housing costs.

Under very limited circumstances, an at-home spouse can obtain an order from a court or an administrative law judge that will allow the at-home spouse to retain income above what would ordinarily be allowed, if the extra income is necessary "due to exceptional circumstances resulting in significant financial duress." For details, the at-home spouse should contact a knowledgeable attorney.

Can an at-home spouse keep additional resources to generate adequate income?

Yes. An at-home spouse can exceed the typical limitations on available resources if the resources are required to generate adequate income for the at-home spouse. An "adequate" income is based on the at-home spouse's income allowance and the related calculations discussed earlier, on pages 60–62. This type of resource increase can be granted only by a court or an administrative law judge.

The rules are most easily explained with an example. Assume that Mrs. Tovar lives in a nursing home and her husband lives in their home. The Tovars have available resources of $150,000. Mrs. Tovar receives a monthly Social Security payment of $1,000, and Mr. Tovar receives a monthly pension of $500. Their state has set a resident's resource allowance of $2,000, a personal needs allowance of $40, an at-home spouse's resource allowance of $90,000, and an at-home spouse's income allowance of $2,260. Mr. Tovar has no excess housing costs.

At first glance, Mrs. Tovar seems to be ineligible for Medicaid because the couple's available resources of $150,000 far exceed their combined resource limit of $92,000 ($90,000 + $2,000). However, because the Tovars' joint income, including interest income, is less than the couple's combined income allowance of $2,300 ($2,260 + $40), the Tovars will be allowed to retain all of their savings. Mr. Tovar needs the additional resources to generate adequate income.

Assume a generous 6 percent simple interest rate on the Tovars' resources. Even with this probably unrealistic interest rate, the Tovars' resources of $150,000 produce $9,000 in interest each year, or $750 monthly. With the interest income added, the Tovars' monthly income totals $2,250—Mrs. Tovar's $1,000 payment plus Mr. Tovar's $500 pension plus the $750 interest.

Because the Tovars' total monthly income of $2,250 is less than the $2,300 total income allowance for the couple ($2,260 for Mr. Tovar, plus $40 for Mrs. Tovar), the Tovars can obtain an order that will increase their resource allowance to a total of $150,000. The increased resource allowance is allowed because it is necessary for the couple to generate adequate income for the at-home spouse.

Couples interested in an increased resource allowance should contact a knowledgeable attorney.

WORD TO THE WISE . . .

This rule protects the frugal. The right to retain additional savings can be useful for couples who have relatively low incomes but significant savings.

After a resident's Medicaid eligibility is established, can the resident be disqualified due to the at-home spouse's increasing resources?
No. Once eligibility is established, the couple must allocate their resources between themselves so that the available resources in the resident's name total no more than the resident's resource allowance (varying from state to state, usually in the vicinity of $2,000). Once this allocation is complete, the resident will remain eligible for Medicaid as long the resident's available resources do not exceed the resident's resource allowance, regardless of the amount of the at-home spouse's available resources.

WORD TO THE WISE . . .

An at-home spouse will not be assessed an undue financial penalty by the resident's need for nursing home care. Once Medicaid eligibility is established, the at-home spouse can retain all monthly income that comes in her name and can retain resources in her name without limitation.

MEDICAID RESOURCE RULES
What resources are considered unavailable by the Medicaid program?
As described in this chapter, the Medicaid program covers only residents with limited resources. Available resources include money, bank accounts, real estate, investments, insurance policies, and other items.

The Medicaid program, however, considers many resources unavailable and will not count those resources against the applicable resource limit. For example, as discussed later, the value of a house used as a residence generally is considered unavailable. The Medicaid program also considers unavailable the value of household goods, a necessary automobile, term life insurance, burial plots, and irrevocable burial plans.

Property used in a business is considered unavailable if the property is used for the support of the resident or the at-home spouse. This exception does not apply to passive investments such as stock purchases.

The cash surrender value of a whole life insurance policy is considered unavailable only if its face value is no more than $1,500. Similarly considered unavailable is a revocable burial plan valued not more than $1,500.

An annuity may be considered unavailable under certain circumstances. On the other hand, resources held in trust for a nursing home resident will generally be considered available to that resident. A detailed discussion of these issues is beyond the scope of this guide; contact a knowledgeable attorney for advice.

Does a nursing home resident have to sell his home to qualify for Medicaid?

Generally not. In most circumstances, a resident's home (his principal residence) is considered an unavailable resource and is not counted against Medicaid resource limitations. For example, the home is considered an unavailable resource if the resident's spouse lives in the home.

Favorable rules apply if the resident's equity in the home is no more than $500,000 or a higher limit set by the state. Such a home is an unavailable resource simply if the resident intends to return to his home. A Medicaid application generally asks the resident if he intends to return to his home; if that question is answered yes, the Medicaid program cannot count the value of the home against the resource limitation, even if the resident has no medically realistic chance of returning to his home.

In thinking about and answering this question, paraphrase the question as "If the resident were to become completely healthy, would the resident live in his home?" If the answer to this paraphrased question is yes, the answer on the Medicaid application also should be yes.

Federal Medicaid law on home ownership was changed in February 2006. For the first time ever, state Medicaid programs are required to consider the amount of an unmarried nursing home resident's home equity. Specifically, a state must deny Medicaid payment for an unmarried nursing home resident if her home equity exceeds $500,000. A state with high home prices may choose to use a higher limit up to $750,000. These two limits—$500,000 and $750,000—will increase slightly in 2011 and subsequent years.

Q & A: KEEPING THE HOME

Q. My father had a massive stroke last month and will most likely have to live in a nursing home for the rest of his life. My mother died three years ago, so my father owns the family home all by himself. He has $400,000 in home equity and $800 in savings. I have legal authority to make financial decisions for my father. Do I have to sell my father's home before he can be eligible for Medicaid?

A. No. Your father will be eligible for Medicaid now, assuming that his Medicaid application is filled out correctly. His home equity of $400,000 is below the limit. On your father's Medicaid application, be sure that you indicate that he intends to return to his home. This would be an accurate answer, because your father would want to return to that house if his condition were to improve.

Some Medicaid eligibility workers mistakenly count a resident's home as an available resource even when the home equity is below the limit. If this happens, contact a knowledgeable attorney for assistance.

As mentioned above, the home equity limits do not apply to married nursing home residents, assuming that the at-home spouse is living in the home in question. The home equity limits also do not apply if the home is occupied by the resident's child and the child is either under age twenty-one or disabled.

It likely will take some time for state Medicaid programs to incorporate this new rule into their procedures, so some states in 2006 or even later may not consider home equity in their application process. Also, there is a slim chance that a court will strike down the new rule due to a procedural mistake made by Congress. In any case, if a resident has too much home equity, she can reduce the equity to the applicable limit by borrowing against the home. Any planning regarding home equity should be done in consultation with a knowledgeable attorney or financial planner.

Although, as discussed, a home generally is considered unavailable, nursing home residents and their representatives are often told to sell the resident's home to pay for nursing home care. This is generally bad advice: such a sale converts an unavailable resource (the home) into an available resource (cash), which will likely make the resident ineligible for Medicaid for an extended period. On rare occasions, a sale is the right choice. More frequently, a sale is made for the wrong reason, because the resident or resident's family does not understand that a home is generally an unavailable resource under Medicaid rules.

Sale of the home is unnecessary even if the resident's home equity exceeds $500,000 or some other higher limit set by the state. The resident is required merely to reduce her home equity to the legal limit, most likely by borrowing against the home. Once the borrowed money is spent down to the Medicaid resident resource allowance, the resident can obtain Medicaid coverage.

A resident's heirs should be aware, however, that a home's special status evaporates after the death of the resident and the resident's spouse (unless an adult disabled child is still living there). As explained on pages 69–70, after a resident's death the Medicaid program may obtain repayment of its expenses from the resident's estate, which in most cases consists primarily of the home.

Are the entire contents of a joint account considered available by the Medicaid program?

In general, yes. The entire contents of a joint account are presumed to be available to a nursing home resident, unless she can clearly trace all or part of the joint account to income or transfers of the other person listed on the joint account.

Can a resident give away resources to become eligible for Medicaid?

In general, no. The Medicaid program looks at any resources given away by the resident in the five years prior to the Medicaid application. If during that time the resident gave away resources for the purpose of making herself Medicaid-eligible, the resident will be ineligible for the amount of time that the given-away resources could have paid for nursing home care.

If, for example, a state's average nursing home rate is $5,000 monthly, a giveaway of $12,500 will cause the resident to be ineligible for two and a half months. The period of ineligibility starts when the resident otherwise would have been eligible.

A giveaway is ignored if it was made more than five years before the month of the resident's Medicaid application. Also ignored are giveaways made to the resident's spouse or disabled child.

The penalty for giveaways does not apply to legitimate purchases, or to gifts that were made for reasons unrelated to Medicaid. For example, a Medicaid penalty will not be assessed for routine gifts made for family members' birthdays or weddings, or for contributions made routinely to the resident's church. On the other hand, a penalty period certainly will be imposed if, for example, the resident gives $100,000 to her adult children and then applies for Medicaid the following month. The general rule is: to avoid a penalty period for a gift, the resident must be able to convince the Medicaid program that the gift was made for reasons unrelated to Medicaid.

These giveaway rules are the result of changes in federal Medicaid law made in February 2006. These changes may not be effective in some states during 2006 and even later. Also, because of a procedural mistake made by Congress, there is a slim chance that a court will strike down the new rule. Nonetheless, anyone even considering the possibility of a giveaway under the "old," less restrictive rules should consult with a knowledgeable attorney before doing anything.

MEDICAID'S RECOVERY FROM DECEASED BENEFICIARY'S ESTATE

After a resident's death, can the Medicaid program take money from the resident's estate to repay the Medicaid program for benefits paid on behalf of the resident?

Yes, in general. The Medicaid claim is limited to the amount of Medicaid payments made on the resident's behalf or the value of the resident's estate, whichever is less.

However, a Medicaid program is prohibited from making a claim if any portion of a resident's property is being passed to a minor or a disabled child. Also, a Medicaid program cannot make a claim against a resident's estate if the resident is survived by a spouse. In some states, the Medicaid program may attempt to trace property that is being passed from the resident to the spouse and then try to collect from the spouse's property after her death.

A Medicaid program must waive an estate claim if the resident's heirs show that enforcement of the claim would cause them to suffer a substantial hardship.

The law pertaining to Medicaid estate claims is complicated and changes frequently. Specific questions should be directed to a knowledgeable attorney.

Can a resident do something now to prevent Medicaid from taking his home after death?

Yes, possibly, depending on the specifics of the situation. This question is beyond the scope of this guide and should be directed to a knowledgeable attorney.

CHAPTER **4**

Admission Process

- Introduction
- Preadmission Requirements
- Admission Agreements
- What If the Nursing Home Says No?

Introduction

Nursing home admissions often occur during stressful times for residents and their family members. In many cases, the process of finding a nursing home has been difficult enough. During the admission process, residents and their families are likely grateful that they found a place and, as a result, may not be inclined to question the nursing home's practices in any way. This can be a serious mistake.

Residents and their families should be aware that problems can arise during the admission process and that the Nursing Home Reform Law contains several protections that apply specifically to the admission process.

This chapter first covers preadmission requirements and then addresses admission agreements. It concludes with a discussion of residents' rights when a nursing home refuses admission.

WORD TO THE WISE . . .

Question staff claims. It's understandable that you may not be comfortable, initially, in questioning some of the claims made by the nursing home staff. Get over it—don't be shy. After reading this guide, you will know more about nursing home law than the average nursing home staff member. Most staff members are not consciously breaking the rules—they simply are doing their jobs in the way that they've been trained and are presenting the contracts and forms that have been given to them by nursing home higher-ups. Let them know when you want something changed or when you see a problem in the admission agreement or some other document.

Preadmission Requirements

Can a nursing home require that a resident pay the private-pay rate for a certain period?

No. The Nursing Home Reform Law requires that a Medicaid-certified nursing home always accept Medicaid, even when a resident has become eligible for Medicaid earlier than the nursing home had anticipated.[1]

This rule is part of a general rule: When a facility is certified for Medicare or Medicaid, the facility must accept that payment as payment in full. The resident can be held liable only for whatever co-payments or deductibles are authorized by Medicare or Medicaid.

Thus, a nursing home cannot require that a resident certify that he is not eligible for Medicare or Medicaid payment of his nursing home expenses. Similarly, a nursing home cannot require a "duration of stay" agreement in which a resident promises that he will pay privately for a certain number of months before utilizing Medicaid benefits.

Can a nursing home require that a resident have a Power of Attorney for Health Care or other type of Health Care Advance Directive?
No. While an advance directive—directing medical decisions in the event of a resident's incapacity and/or appointing an agent to make health care decisions—is useful for every resident, it cannot be required as a condition of admission.

More information on advance directives is available in chapter 7 of this guide.

Can a nursing home require that a resident post a deposit as a condition of admission?
A nursing home cannot require a deposit from a resident if either the Medicare program or the Medicaid program makes payments for the resident's stay in the nursing home. This is true even if the nursing home claims that the money is advance payment of required Medicare co-payments.

A nursing home may, however, require a deposit from a resident who pays for her stay in the nursing home without assistance from the Medicaid or Medicare programs.

Admission Agreements

Residents and family members may be inclined to sign any document that the nursing home presents and accept whatever conditions the nursing home sets, but this inclination should be resisted. Some nursing homes knowingly or unknowingly include in their admission agreements provisions that are unfair or even illegal. If these conditions are accepted, the admission agreement may come back to haunt the residents and their families.

This section first covers general issues relating to admission agreements; it then discusses the financial liability of family members or friends and examines the inappropriateness of arbitration provisions.

Who signs an admission agreement if the incoming resident is mentally incapacitated?

Alzheimer's disease and similar dementias are common among nursing home residents. When an incoming resident is unable to understand and enter into a contract because of a mental incapacity, the nursing home may ask a representative to sign in the resident's place. Ideally, the representative will be someone with explicit legal authority to make decisions for the resident—for example, an agent appointed through a power of attorney.

Unfortunately, more often than not, the incoming resident had not taken the necessary steps to appoint a legal representative when she still had the legal capacity to do so. Nursing homes will usually then ask a family member—often the resident's adult child—to sign as the resident's representative, even though the family member has no explicit legal authority to make decisions for the resident.

Without formal delegated powers—through a power of attorney, for example—the family member's authority to sign on the resident's behalf is a bit shaky. Nonetheless, in most cases it is acceptable for the family member to sign, just to keep the process moving. However, the family member should be careful not to sign as "guarantor" or "responsible party," because such a signature can likely be used by the nursing home to argue that the fam-

---

WORD TO THE WISE . . .

Plan ahead. All of us are vulnerable to Alzheimer's disease, stroke, and other conditions. Advance planning—for example, appointing an agent through a power-of-attorney document—can make life easier for both you and your family.

ily member is personally liable for all nursing home expenses. This issue of third-party financial liability is discussed on pages 78–83 of this guide.

How can residents and their family members recognize problems in an admission agreement before the agreement is signed?

Too often, admission agreement terms are illegal and biased in the nursing home's favor. A resident and his family should look at the agreement carefully and watch for illegal or unfair terms. Such provisions should be deleted whenever possible.

Deletion of illegal or unfair terms is much easier if the resident has already moved into the nursing home. Once the resident has moved in, he has much greater leverage. As explained in the section on evictions (see chapter 8), a nursing home can force a resident to move only for certain specified reasons. A nursing home

YOU CAN DO IT!

It may be difficult to point out to a nursing home staff member that the admission agreement contains illegal or unfair terms. But the alternative is worse—accepting illegal or unfair terms that may be enforced against the resident.

This is an issue that comes up over and over again in dealing with a nursing home—is it better to point out problems or to stay silent? This guide generally follows the principle that the squeaky wheel gets the grease. When you're being wronged, you should complain—intelligently and persistently. If you're right, do not accept no for an answer. On the other hand, when the nursing home care is particularly thoughtful, you should thank the appropriate staff members.

cannot evict a resident for the resident's (or representative's) deletion of illegal or unfair terms from the contract.

If the nursing home requires that the admission agreement be signed before the resident enters the facility, the leverage of the resident and his family is reduced but not eliminated. This guide recommends that the resident or family member examine the admission agreement carefully and then politely but firmly request deletion of any illegal or unfair terms. More often than not, the nursing home will comply to avoid any more attention being placed on the offending terms.

What problems should a resident look out for in an admission agreement?

The following are some common problems in nursing home admission agreements.

Making a Family Member or Friend Liable for All Nursing Home Expenses *Problem.* Admission agreement says that a family member or friend will be personally liable for all nursing home charges. The federal Nursing Home Reform Law prohibits a nursing home from requiring such financial guarantees. See pages 78–83 for more detail.

Requiring Arbitration of Disputes *Problem.* Admission agreement refers all future disputes between the resident and the nursing home to a private arbitrator rather than the court system. Arbitration terms are often unfair to residents. See pages 83–85 for more detail.

Authorizing Illegal Discharges *Problem.* Admission agreement includes eviction justifications beyond those allowed by the

Nursing Home Reform Law. See chapter 8 for discussion of the evictions allowed by the reform law.

Limiting Resident's Right to Be Readmitted *Problem.* Admission agreement limits the right of a Medicaid-eligible resident to be readmitted after a hospital stay. See pages 159–64 for discussion of the right of a Medicaid-eligible resident to be readmitted to the nursing home after a hospital stay of any length.

Limiting Resident's Right to Refuse Transfer from Medicare-Certified Bed *Problem.* Admission agreement provision limits the resident's rights under the Nursing Home Reform Law to refuse transfer from a Medicare-certified bed. See pages 163–65 for more information on this right.

Waiving Nursing Home's Responsibility *Problem.* Admission agreement says that the resident is completely or partially releasing the nursing home from responsibility for the resident's health or belongings. These waivers of liability are generally illegal and unenforceable under contract law, which prohibits enforcement of liability waivers when consumers' well-being is involved.

WORD TO THE WISE . . .

Get a copy. Be absolutely sure that you get and retain a copy of the admission agreement. When possible, do not have anyone sign it until the resident has moved in. Do not let the nursing home rush the signature process.

FINANCIAL LIABILITY OF FAMILY MEMBERS OR FRIENDS

Can a nursing home require that a resident's family member or friend become personally liable for the nursing home's bills?

No. The Nursing Home Reform Law prohibits a nursing home from requiring a third-party guarantee of payment as a condition of a resident's admission or continued stay.[2] Thus, a resident's family member or friend cannot be required to guarantee the resident's payments to a nursing home.

However, a nursing home can ask a person who has legal control over the resident's money to sign the contract as the resident's representative. In this case, the signer obligates only the resident's money, not his own.

Why does the reform law prohibit financial guarantees? Car dealers, for example, often require that a buyer have a cosigner. Why shouldn't nursing homes have the same right?

The no-financial-guarantee rule of the reform law is supported by at least three reasons. First, because Medicaid pays for nursing home care for residents in financial need, the nursing home is already protected if the resident runs out of money. By contrast, if a car buyer runs out of money, he will be unable to make his payments, and the car dealer will have to look to a guarantor for payment.

Second, a financial guarantee of nursing home expenses exposes the guarantor to unlimited liability—maybe $10,000 or $50,000 or even $100,000, depending on how many months of nursing home care are at issue. A financial guarantor for a car purchase, of course, can be liable for no more than the cost of the car.

Third, a nursing home can hold tremendous leverage over a family if the prospective resident needs a nursing home immediately and has relatively few options. The no-financial-guarantee rule gives some protection to prospective residents and families who may feel as though the nursing home has them over a barrel in the discussion of the terms of admission.

What is the significance of signing an admission agreement as a "responsible party"?

The phrase "responsible party" is used by some nursing homes in an attempt to evade the reform law's no-financial-guarantee rule. The agreements ask for the signature of a "responsible party." In most cases, family members and friends routinely sign on the "responsible party" signature line, assuming that the "responsible party" is a designated contact person. The family member or friend signs as "responsible party" because he or she wants to be consulted on the resident's care in the nursing home and notified of any issues or problems.

What the family member or friend may not realize is that "responsible party" is typically defined in the middle of the admission agreement as a person who is financially liable for any and all nursing home expenses. Generally, the admission agreement even recites that the "responsible party" has volunteered to take on financial responsibility.

Of course, this claim of volunteering is nonsense. There is no reason why any rational person would volunteer to take on financial liability when the reform law specifically says that a nursing home is prohibited from requiring financial guarantees.

These admission agreements are written to trick family members and friends into signing as responsible parties. If a problem ever develops with a resident's account, the nursing home will undoubtedly try to require the "responsible party" to pay the disputed amount personally. If the "responsible party" then points out that the reform law prohibits third-party financial guarantees, the nursing home will claim that the reform law does not apply, because the family member or friend supposedly volunteered to become financially responsible.

What should a family member or friend do if she is asked to sign as a "responsible party" or become financially liable for the resident's nursing home care in some other way?

Just say no. No family member or friend should agree to become financially responsible for a resident's nursing home bills. Such an agreement cannot be required and legally offers no benefit to a resident.

If the family member or friend refuses to take on financial responsibility, won't the nursing home retaliate by refusing to admit the prospective resident?

Without a doubt, saying no is easier when the resident already has moved into the nursing home. At that point, the family member can refuse to sign as a "responsible party" with little or no risk. As explained in the section on evictions (see chapter 8), a nursing home can force a resident to leave only for certain, limited reasons. The refusal of a family member or friend to become financially responsible is certainly not one of those reasons. Remember, the reform law prohibits a nursing home from requiring a financial guarantee.

Things are a bit trickier when the resident has not yet moved into the nursing home. On occasion, a nursing home will not accept an individual until the admission agreement—including the "responsible party" signature line—is signed. In this situation, the family member or friend has two choices: one, refuse to sign as a "responsible party" or, two, sign as a "responsible party" and hope that the "responsible party" provision never is enforced.

This guide recommends the first choice. The family member or friend should politely but firmly explain that financial guarantees cannot be required and for that reason decline to sign as a "responsible party." More often than not, the nursing home staff

> **WORD TO THE WISE . . .**
>
> *Point out flaws in contracts.* Don't be embarrassed to point out to the nursing home staff member that "responsible party" provisions are illegal. It is the nursing home that should be embarrassed by its attempted evasion of the reform law.

member will concede the point and continue processing the admission.

Can anything be done for a family member or friend who has already signed a financial guarantee?

Yes. A "responsible party" financial guarantee is unenforceable for at least three reasons.

First, even though the admission agreement claims that the "responsible party" has volunteered to become financially responsible, the nursing home has, in reality, required the financial guarantee. The nursing home staff member has likely told the family member or friend to sign as a "responsible party," oftentimes by placing a big *X* in front of the "responsible party" signature line. Because the nursing home has required the financial guarantee, the nursing home has violated the Nursing Home Reform Law, and the financial guarantee is illegal.

Second, a "responsible party" financial guarantee is illegally deceptive. As discussed, a family member generally signs as a "responsible party" while believing that no financial liability is involved and that a "responsible party" is merely a contact person.

Third, the financial guarantee is unenforceable under basic contract law rules because it does not benefit either the resident or the "responsible party." The only possible benefit would be if signing the financial guarantee were needed to arrange or accelerate

A SHORT INTRODUCTION TO CONTRACT LAW

A gratuitous promise is one that does not involve a return benefit. Gratuitous promises are unenforceable in court.

Here's an example. If John Doe promises to pay you $10,000 for your car and then fails to do so, you could have a viable contract case against Mr. Doe. On the other hand, if Mr. Doe promises to give you $10,000 for your birthday and then fails to do so, you will not have a case.

Courts don't waste their time enforcing gratuitous promises like Mr. Doe's birthday promise. Likewise, a court will not enforce a financial guarantee for nursing home expenses that states that the "responsible party" is not required to take on financial liability but has volunteered to take on such liability. Neither the resident nor the "responsible party" receives a benefit from such a financial guarantee, so the promise is unenforceable.

the resident's admission—but the reform law specifically states that admission to a nursing home cannot be dependent in any way on the signing of a financial guarantee.

If a nursing home threatens to enforce a financial guarantee, the threatened family member or friend should immediately contact a knowledgeable attorney.

Can a nursing home require a resident's representative to agree to apply the resident's money to nursing home charges?

Yes. Notwithstanding the preceding discussion about financial guarantees, a nursing home may require a resident's representative—for example, a conservator or guardian, a Medicaid representative, a representative payee for Social Security benefits, an agent under a financial power of attorney—to agree to apply the resident's money to nursing home charges. As discussed, a resident's authorized representative cannot be required to guarantee payment with the representative's own money.

Should a nursing home admission agreement include a promise by a resident's representative to take all necessary steps to have the nursing home charges paid?
No. Here, too, the nursing home would be attempting to evade the Nursing Home Reform Law's no-financial-guarantee rule. This language is effectively equivalent to a financial guarantee. If payment on the resident's account falls behind for any reason, the nursing home will improperly claim the right to payment from both the resident and the representative.

Is the resident's representative financially liable to the nursing home if the representative steals the resident's money rather than uses it to pay the nursing home?
The representative might be liable to the nursing home, but there is no need for any specific language in the admission agreement.

Under a standard legal rule, the representative's legal obligation is to the resident, not the nursing home. However, an exception is made if the representative has committed a crime. If the representative has stolen from the resident rather than paid the nursing home, the representative has committed a crime and as a result can be financially liable to the nursing home.

ARBITRATION
What is a binding arbitration agreement?
Arbitration is a decision-making process in which disputes are decided by a private arbitrator rather than by a judge or jury.

In a binding arbitration agreement, the decision of the arbitrator is final and cannot be appealed to any court. If a nursing home resident signs an admission agreement with a binding arbitration clause, the resident is committed to arbitration even if he

A COMMON PROBLEM: DELAY IN MEDICAID ELIGIBILITY

Many nonpayment situations in a nursing home result from a delay in the resident's Medicaid eligibility. The delay might be due to mistakes made by the resident, the resident's representative, the nursing home, or the Medicaid program. As discussed, the representative should not be held personally liable.

One often-overlooked strategy is to have the resident's monthly Medicaid patient pay amount designated to the past-due bill rather than the current month's charges. Designating the patient pay amount to the old bill will pay down the old bill and, since the patient pay amount has already been paid, the Medicaid program will pay the entire current month's bill.

Assume, for example, that a resident has a past-due bill of $10,000 and a monthly Medicaid patient pay amount of $1,000. The patient pay amount should be applied to the past-due bill, which allows the Medicaid program to pay all of the current month's bill. In ten months, the past-due bill will be paid off in full.

Additional information on this strategy is available in the Medicaid section, on pages 52–53.

realizes afterward that arbitration was a bad choice. If a resident has a claim against the nursing home for poor care, for example, a lawsuit by the resident against the nursing home must be resolved through arbitration rather than court procedures.

As discussed in the following section, a resident may be able to escape a binding arbitration clause if he can show that he was deceived into signing the arbitration clause or if requiring arbitration would be grossly unfair. However, the situation can best be avoided by refusing to sign such a clause in the first place.

Should a resident or a resident's representative agree to arbitration in an admission agreement?

No. There is no need to commit to arbitration during the admission process. If arbitration is really the best option, the resident can make that choice knowledgeably after the particular dispute has arisen and after she has had an opportunity to consult with an attorney.

During admission, however, the resident doesn't know what type of dispute may arise between her and the nursing home and, most likely, isn't thinking about disputes and arbitration at all. She is probably overwhelmed by the reality of moving into a nursing home.

Another factor against arbitration is the fact that the arbitration process may be biased in favor of the nursing home. For example, the chosen arbitrator may tend to favor nursing homes in disputes against residents, or the arbitration agreement may limit the remedies available to residents. Residents generally fare better in the court system, with jury trials, than in arbitration.

Finally, arbitration can be expensive. An arbitrator may charge several thousand dollars a day, often with the cost split between the resident and the nursing home.

If a resident or a resident's representative has already signed an admission agreement with an arbitration provision, must all disputes with the nursing home be handled through arbitration?

Not necessarily. The arbitration provision may be unenforceable because it is grossly unfair or because of some other legal reason. The resident should contact a knowledgeable attorney to discuss the situation.

What If the Nursing Home Says No?

As discussed in chapter 2, a person needing nursing home care should look at potential nursing homes carefully. But the choosing process is a two-way street—the resident chooses the nursing home, but then the nursing home must be willing to admit the resident.

If a nursing home has few or no vacancies, it can afford to be selective in the applicants that it admits. On the other hand, if a nursing home has a high vacancy rate, the nursing home is more likely to admit virtually any applicant.

Does a nursing home have to accept every person who wants to be admitted?

No. In general, a nursing home can choose whether to reject or accept any particular applicant. In some cases, however, a facility's rejection of an applicant is illegal discrimination. As this guide discusses, the most common types of discrimination are those against applicants who are Medicaid-eligible or have relatively difficult or disagreeable health conditions.

Can a nursing home refuse to admit an applicant because he is eligible for Medicaid?

Nursing homes have a love-hate relationship with Medicaid reimbursement. They love it because roughly two-thirds of nursing home residents are Medicaid-eligible. They hate it because the Medicaid rate is generally the lowest reimbursement rate— substantially less than either the Medicare rate or the private-pay rate.

For most nursing homes, accepting Medicaid is a business necessity. Because so many nursing home residents are Medicaid-eligible, 94 percent of nursing homes nationwide are certified to accept Medicaid.

Because Medicaid reimbursement rates are comparatively low, many nursing homes try to keep their Medicaid-eligible residents to no more than a certain percentage of the facility population. As discussed on pages 152–53, some states allow a nursing home to certify only a certain number of its beds for Medicaid. In the other states, a Medicaid-certified nursing home is required to certify all of its beds for Medicaid, although in these states a nursing home is likely to try to limit its percentage of Medicaid-eligible residents by rejecting Medicaid-eligible applicants.

As a practical matter, federal law provides little protection for a Medicaid-eligible applicant who has been rejected by a nursing home that had a Medicaid-certified bed available when the application was made. Nursing homes are not required to give a reason for rejecting an applicant. Furthermore, as discussed, a nursing home generally has discretion to admit or reject applicants.

A few states have laws that prohibit or limit discrimination against Medicaid-eligible applicants:

- In Connecticut, a nursing home must admit applicants on a first-come, first-serve basis unless the nursing home's Medicaid-eligible population is already 70 percent or more of the nursing home's total residents.[3]
- Massachusetts and North Dakota explicitly prohibit discrimination against Medicaid-eligible applicants.[4]
- Minnesota requires that the private-pay rate not exceed the Medicaid daily rate so that a nursing home will not have an incentive to prefer a private-pay applicant over a Medicaid-eligible applicant.[5]
- New Jersey requires Medicaid-eligible applicants to be admitted as they reach the top of a nursing home's waiting list, until the nursing home's percentage of Medicaid-eligible residents is equal to or greater than the statewide average.[6]
- New York requires that a nursing home admit a "reasonable percentage" of Medicaid-eligible applicants.[7]
- Ohio does not allow a nursing home to discriminate based on Medicaid eligibility unless 80 percent or more of the nursing home's residents are already Medicaid-eligible.[8]

Can a nursing home refuse to admit an applicant because she is likely to become eligible for Medicaid in the near future?

Nursing homes commonly ask an applicant for information regarding her income and savings. With this information, a nursing home can estimate with relative ease when the applicant will spend down her savings to the point where she will be Medicaid-eligible.

Federal law does not explicitly prohibit a nursing home from requiring such financial disclosure. The most relevant federal law (discussed in detail on p. 72) is the prohibition against duration-of-stay agreements. Under this prohibition, an applicant or resident cannot be required to promise that she will pay the private-pay rate (i.e., not become Medicaid-eligible) through at least a specific month.

Under certain circumstances, a nursing home's financial disclosure requirements could be challenged by characterizing them as being equivalent to a duration-of-stay agreement. By requiring financial disclosure, as in requiring a duration-of-stay agreement, the nursing home is taking steps to ensure that the resident will not use Medicaid until a particular month.

Can a nursing home reject an applicant because he has a relatively difficult or disagreeable health condition?

In general, nursing homes tend to prefer applicants with routine, straightforward care needs. An applicant with higher-than-average care needs may have a difficult time finding a nursing home willing to admit him, even if (as is likely) the care needs are within the type of care that by law nursing homes must be capable of providing.

Discrimination against those with higher care needs is a violation of federal antidiscrimination law, including the Americans with Disabilities Act. In one case, a federal appeals court ruled that a nursing home was obligated by federal antidiscrimination law to admit a woman with combative behavior caused by the progression of Alzheimer's disease. Before the court order, the nursing home's refusal to admit the woman had forced her to stay in a nursing home approximately eighty-five miles from her husband and children.[9]

Applicants who are denied admission based on health care needs may wish to consult a knowledgeable attorney about possible options. Note, however, that few cases are brought against nursing homes for discriminating against an applicant based on the applicant's care needs. Most applicants find it easier and more time effective to look for another nursing home rather than contest one nursing home's refusal to admit.

Currently, discrimination based on an applicant's health care needs is common among nursing homes across the country. This state of affairs could be improved if more applicants were to challenge denials under the federal antidiscrimination law.

Can a nursing home reject an applicant because she doesn't speak English?

No. Under federal civil rights law, a nursing home that receives federal funds (such as Medicare or Medicaid reimbursement) cannot discriminate against individuals based on national origin, race, or color.[10] Discrimination based on national origin includes denying services or giving different care to individuals who don't speak English.

An applicant denied nursing home admission because of language should file a complaint with her regional Office of Civil Rights of the U.S. Department of Health and Human Services. She may also wish to consult with a knowledgeable attorney about her rights and options.

Notes

1. Section 483.12(d)(1) of Title 42 of the Code of Federal Regulations states that a nursing home cannot require a resident to waive any current or future right to Medicare or Medicaid reimbursement.

2. The provision prohibiting a nursing home from requiring a third-party guarantee of payment is located at section 483.12(d)(2) of Title 42 of the Code of Federal Regulations.

3. This law (with additional exceptions) can be found at section 19a-533 of the Connecticut statutes, and at section 17-311-209 of the Connecticut regulations.

4. This law can be found at section 4.03(1) of Title 940 of the Massachusetts regulations, and section 50-10.2-02(1)(r) of the North Dakota statutes.

5. This law can be found at section 256B.48(a) of the Minnesota statutes.

6. This law can be found at section 10:5-12.2 of the New Jersey statutes and section 8:39-5.2(a)(2) of Title 8 of the New Jersey regulations.

7. This law can be found at section 670.3(c)(2) of Title 10 of the New York regulations.

8. This law can be found at section 5111.31(A)(4) of the Ohio statutes.

9. The case discussed is *Wagner v. Fair Acres Geriatric Center*, decided by the federal Third Circuit Court of Appeals in 1995. The citation for this case is 49 F.3d 1002 (3rd Cir. 1995).

10. This antidiscrimination law can be found at section 2000d of Title 42 of the United States Code.

5

Moving In

- Introduction
- Moving to a Nursing Home
- Making the Transition
- Safeguarding Residents' Property

Introduction

The move to a nursing home is a major adjustment. This chapter discusses the move to the nursing home, the subsequent transition period, and the law that applies to safeguarding residents' property.

Moving to a Nursing Home

How can the resident and family prepare for the move to a nursing home?

Moving is one of the most stressful events in life. Moving to a nursing home can be particularly anxiety provoking.

Ideally, the resident should visit the nursing home once or twice before moving in. The move will be somewhat easier if the resident recognizes at least a few faces on the staff or has gotten acquainted with her roommate.

In preparing for a move to a nursing home, the more planning, the better. It is preferable to plan what will happen rather than avoid the topic and hope that details will work themselves out. Planning should address both logistics and emotions.

The extent and type of planning will depend to a certain extent on the health and personality of the individual entering the nursing home and the family dynamics. Ideally, the resident and the family will be willing and able to discuss the next steps.

A resident and her family can benefit from an honest discussion of fears and concerns. The resident is facing many changes. She is leaving a home and neighborhood in exchange for a shared living space that will not likely feel very homey and may feel some-

---

WORD TO THE WISE . . .

Moving can be a challenge. The move to a nursing home is often traumatic for both resident and family. In many cases, this guide's recommendations are much easier said than done, particularly if the need for a nursing home arises suddenly.

The resident or a family member may be in denial about the need for a nursing home. The resident's adult children may be in conflict. Family members may feel as though they've let the resident down, by not being able to take care of the resident at home or by living in another state.

Do the best that you can. And if the move feels painful or the family conversations were not quite as satisfying as they could have been, don't beat yourself up. You are facing practical problems and emotional issues that don't lend themselves to easy solutions.

what institutional. More often than not, the resident will be sharing a room with a resident whom she does not know.

The move to the nursing home is also difficult for family members—for a resident's spouse, of course, but also for children, grandchildren, and others. Family members can benefit from discussion with the resident and with one another.

What should the resident bring with him?

The resident will need to bring clothes, jackets, and shoes, along with combs, toothbrushes, and other toiletries. In addition, the resident has the right under the federal Nursing Home Reform Law to bring other personal possessions to the extent possible. The relevant federal regulation states that each "resident has the right to retain and use personal possessions, including some furnishings, and appropriate clothing, as space permits, unless to do so would infringe upon the rights or health and safety of other residents."[1]

As a practical matter, a resident's right to bring personal possessions is limited by the size of most nursing home rooms. In a shared room, a resident may have as little as eighty square feet—for example, a space eight feet by ten feet. A bed, chair, and table can easily take up all or most of a resident's allotted space.

On the other hand, many personal possessions are not particularly large, and they should fit easily within a nursing home room. Pictures and other mementos are good examples. Nursing home rooms often have corkboards so that residents can post pictures on the wall.

Clocks, radios, calendars, books, magazines—all of these can be accommodated with little difficulty. Televisions are common, and computers are occasionally seen in nursing home rooms.

Individual nursing homes may have policies that limit a resident's right to bring in personal possessions. These policies should be compared to the federal regulation that allows a resident to bring in personal possessions as long as they do not violate other

---

WORD TO THE WISE . . .

Don't give up. Stand your ground if the nursing home claims that a particular personal possession is not allowed. Point out to the nursing home that the federal law approves personal possessions at the nursing home unless other residents' rights, health, or safety are affected.

---

residents' rights, health, or safety. The regulation prevails—regardless of a nursing home's policy, a resident has the right to bring in any possession that does not infringe upon other residents' rights, health, or safety.

To the extent possible, the resident's name should be put on everything. For clothing, either the resident's name should be written with waterproof marker, or a name tag should be sewn into the clothes.

Should a resident bring valuables to the nursing home?

This guide suggests that a resident generally not bring valuables to the nursing home.

One very real concern is the possibility that a valuable item—most likely, jewelry—will be lost or stolen. Expensive items disappear all the time in nursing homes, and oftentimes it is unclear whether the fault lies with the resident or the nursing home. And as a practical matter, even if the resident or resident's family is convinced that the nursing home is at fault, the nursing home will not likely volunteer to pay the resident for the value of the missing item. The nursing home will not likely take responsibility unless it is found at fault by state inspectors or a small-claims court.

Ultimately, it is the resident's choice whether to bring valuables into a nursing home. Is the comfort of a treasured item of jewelry worth the risk that it may be lost? Residents and families should understand that the risk is real. One alternative is to have the nursing home keep the expensive item locked up in an office. Another alternative is to have the item kept by a family member and brought to the resident on occasion.

If a valuable item is lost or stolen at a nursing home, the nursing home may be responsible. Establishing the nursing home's responsibility is difficult (as discussed) but not impossible.

Can a resident or resident's family set up a video camera to record care of the resident?

Yes, although the nursing home likely will object.

Videotaping is increasingly common in the United States. Many retail stores routinely videotape anyone who enters or exits. Some preschools use video cameras to record daily activities, allowing parents to look in at any time through the Internet.

For peace of mind, some family members of nursing home residents would like to use video cameras to record the goings-on in the resident's room. Frequently, because of dementia of one type or another, nursing home residents are unable to describe what happens to them or how care has been provided or not provided. Videotaping allows family members to see what happens in a resident's room. Also, the presence of a video camera keeps the nursing home staff on its toes. The presence of a camera is a good way to prevent residents from being ignored or abused.

Use of a video camera in most cases is relatively easy. Usually, a family member changes the videotape as necessary and then reviews the tape to make sure that nothing improper has occurred.

A few nursing homes invite families to set up video cameras in residents' rooms, but these nursing homes are the exception. Most nursing homes actively oppose use of video cameras in residents' rooms, arguing that the cameras violate the privacy of residents and staff members and complaining that the use of cameras is designed to support abuse lawsuits against nursing homes.

The nursing homes' privacy concerns can be addressed. Before using a video camera in a resident's room, the resident's family should have the consent of the resident and the resident's roommate. If the resident or roommate is not mentally competent, the consent of the appropriate representative is necessary.

Possibly, any invasion of the roommate's privacy could be reduced or eliminated by keeping the camera pointed far away from the roommate's half of the room and by not recording any sound. Nonetheless, the better alternative is to obtain the consent of the roommate or the roommate's representative.

Consent of staff members is not needed, because videotaping does not violate their privacy. They are performing their jobs in full view of residents and others. Just as convenience store clerks, for example, are videotaped while working, nursing home staff members also can be videotaped. A sign in the resident's room should notify staff members that videotaping is taking place.

Regarding nursing homes' arguments that videotaping is designed to support lawsuits, it should be noted that videotaping is most effective as a deterrent. Videotaping should be open, not secret, so that the nursing home staff is more likely to provide good care, and abuse is prevented.

Currently, the laws of only two states—New Mexico and Texas—explicitly recognize the right of a resident's family to place a video camera in a resident's room. In these states, a particular process must be followed to ensure that the roommate (or the roommate's representative) has consented and that anyone who enters the resident's room is aware that videotaping is taking place.

In other states, the nursing home is likely to object. This guide recommends that residents or family members consult with a knowledgeable attorney but consider primarily the strategy of openly installing the video camera and forcing the nursing home to respond. If the resident and the roommate consent to the camera's presence and if notification of the taping is posted conspicuously in the resident's room, the nursing home should have no legitimate reason for complaint.

Making the Transition

How can the family help the resident adjust to the nursing home?

It's common sense: Family members and friends should visit whenever possible. Visits are great for the resident, and they help to ensure that the nursing home gives adequate attention to the resident—that is, visitors can make sure that the staff meets the resident's needs. Also, visitors can help by becoming acquainted with the staff members who care for the resident. Personal relationships with staff go a long way in ensuring that the resident's care is up to par.

If, while at home, the incoming nursing home resident had been assisted by an aide, the aide should periodically visit the resident for at least the first few weeks of the resident's stay in the nursing home. Of course, money is an issue—the resident or family first has to determine if continuing payment to the aide is financially possible and justified.

When can a nursing home resident receive visitors?

A resident's family member must generally be allowed to visit the resident at any time, assuming that the resident wishes to be visited by that family member at that time. Similarly, a resident's friend must generally be allowed to visit the resident if the resident wishes to receive such a visit, although a nursing home can set reasonable visiting hours for social visits from persons who are not family members.

A representative from the Long-Term Care Ombudsman program must generally be allowed to visit the resident at any time

---

Q & A: VISITING HOURS

Q. My son works until 7:00 PM, and wants to visit me at 8:00 PM. The nursing home says that visiting hours end at 7:30 PM. Can my son visit me after 7:30 PM?

A. Yes. A resident's right to visit with family members cannot be limited by a nursing home's visiting hours.

(see pp. 172–73 for more about this program). The same rules apply to a resident's doctor. An individual who provides the resident with health, social, or legal services—a therapist, for example—must be given reasonable access to the resident, assuming that the resident wishes to see that individual.

Can a nursing home bar a visitor whom the nursing home staff considers unlikable or bothersome?

Generally not. As explained, a resident has a right to see a visitor. The resident's right is only meaningful if it trumps a nursing home's desire to keep the visitor out. In general, a nursing home can turn away a visitor only at the request of the resident or the resident's legal representative, or if the nursing home has obtained a court order that bars the visitor. Such a court order could be granted only in extreme and unusual circumstances, given a resident's right to receive visitors.

WORD TO THE WISE . . .

Visit at off-hours. Consider visiting the nursing home late at night or before the sun rises, to make sure that the overnight employees are providing proper care.

WORD TO THE WISE . . .

Visitors are a resident's choice. Disputes over visitors are not uncommon. Sometimes a family member thinks that visits from another family member are disruptive and wants the nursing home to keep that person out. At other times, it is the nursing home itself that wants to bar a particular visitor. The key thing to remember is that the decision rests with the resident or the resident's legal representative. Unless the family member is the legal representative, that family member does not have authority to bar a particular visitor. The nursing home also does not have such authority.

If the family member or nursing home wants a particular visitor to be barred, the only option is to obtain a court order. It should be noted, however, that in most cases a court will refuse to grant such an order, based on the resident's right to receive visitors.

How can family members ensure that a resident's particular needs, wishes, and habits are known and respected by nursing home staff members?

It may be helpful for the family to write down information about the resident's key needs, wishes, and habits and then post that information in the resident's room. The information may include preferred sleeping and eating patterns (early riser or night owl?), favorite activities (walks, special television shows), special dietary needs and preferences, and religious practices, as well as any other information that would be helpful for staff to know.

These needs, wishes, and habits should also be identified during the resident's assessment and then taken into account in the resident's care plan. The family should actively participate in developing the care plan, as discussed on pages 113–14.

Family members should talk to the nursing home staff members and, if possible, be friendly with them. At a minimum, family members should learn the names of the staff members who work with the resident and develop some sort of personal relationship with those staff members.

Safeguarding Residents' Property

Nursing home residents often may not have the physical or mental strength to safeguard their own property. As a result, the possession and management of residents' property can create a range of potential problems. Applicable law determines if a nursing home can demand control of a resident's property, what a nursing home must do with resident property specifically entrusted to it, and what a nursing home must do to protect resident property not specifically entrusted to the nursing home.

Can a resident be required to deposit her personal funds with a nursing home?

No. This practice is prohibited by the Nursing Home Reform Law. A resident has the right to manage her own financial affairs.

Can a resident require a nursing home to hold and safeguard the resident's personal funds or property?

Yes. The reform law requires that nursing homes offer this service. If a resident or resident's representative makes a written request that the nursing home hold the resident's money, the nursing home must do so.

What must a nursing home do with a resident's funds or property that the nursing home has agreed to hold and safeguard?

A nursing home must deposit all resident funds over $50 into an interest-bearing account that is separate from the nursing home's operating account. Any interest accrued must be attributed properly to the resident's account.

To ensure that these procedures are followed, a nursing home must maintain an accounting of each resident's funds and a written record of each transaction involving those funds. The nursing home must allow a resident to review these financial records.

Must a nursing home take any steps to safeguard a resident's property not specifically entrusted to the nursing home?
Yes. All nursing homes must develop a policy that prevents theft or misappropriation of a resident's property. Any allegations of misappropriation must be investigated and reported to nursing home management and to the appropriate authorities.

WORD TO THE WISE . . .

Watch your valuables. Residents should keep a list of all of their property kept at the nursing home. If at all possible, they should not keep irreplaceable or valuable items at the nursing home. Resident property is commonly lost and stolen. The nursing home may be liable, depending on whether it failed to take adequate steps to protect or monitor the property.

Note

1. This regulation is found at section 483.10(l) of Title 42 of the Code of Federal Regulations.

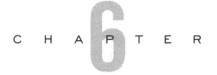

C H A P T E R **6**

Quality of Care

- Introduction
- Basic Principles
- Making Choices and Planning for Care
- General Care
- Medical Conditions
- Access to Medical Services and Medications
- Minimizing Use of Physical and Chemical Restraints
- Meals and Schedules
- Staffing Requirements

Introduction

The Nursing Home Reform Law sets a high standard for nursing home quality of care. The reform law's foundation is as follows: "Each resident must receive and the facility must provide the necessary care and services to attain or maintain the highest practicable physical, mental, and psychosocial well-being."[1] This requirement of the reform law protects every resident of any nursing home that is certified to accept reimbursement from the Medicare or Medicaid programs, whether or not the care of the individual resident is reimbursed through Medicare or Medicaid.

The quality of care provided by a nursing home depends on a variety of factors. For example, the care received by a resident depends in part on the qualifications of the staff and the sophistication of the medical equipment. In addition, a resident's care depends on less-measurable considerations, such as the diligence of the staff and the nursing home's general atmosphere.

As discussed in this chapter, the reform law sets many standards designed to ensure good quality of care. For example, it requires assessments, care planning, nurse staffing, and staff training.

Residents and family members should be prepared to improve a nursing home's quality of care by insisting on the nursing home's compliance with relevant laws and regulations. On questions concerning quality of care, residents and family members too frequently defer to a nursing home, assuming that laypersons shouldn't dabble in medical issues.

Residents and family members are actually well able to make decisions regarding the resident's care. Many issues relating to quality of care involve little technical information: A nursing home generally falls short not because it makes a bad treatment decision but

---

WORD TO THE WISE . . .

Services must enable residents to reach the highest possible level of functioning. If you remember nothing else about the reform law, remember that each nursing home is obligated to provide a resident with the care necessary for the resident to reach or remain at the highest level of functioning. This is a simple and important rule that is relevant in virtually every situation involving a resident's care.

because its staff members fail to perform necessary tasks. Informed pressure applied by residents and family members can cause a nursing home to hire more staff members or demand better performance from the existing staff.

This chapter covers basic principles, planning for care, general care, specific medical conditions, access to medications and services, meals and schedules, and staffing requirements.

Basic Principles

Must a nursing home help a resident to improve his condition?

Yes, to the extent possible. Under the Nursing Home Reform Law, as quoted, "each resident must receive and the facility must provide the necessary care and services to attain or maintain the highest practicable physical, mental, and psychosocial well-being." In general, this requirement means that a resident's condition should not decline in a nursing home unless the resident's condition makes such a decline inevitable. As the term suggests, the nursing home is expected to *nurse* the resident to improved health to the extent possible.

A resident may need specific therapy treatments to regain function. If the resident's doctor prescribes the therapy, the nursing home must ensure that the therapy is provided.

In many cases, however, the resident's doctor is the sticking point in obtaining therapy. Often, the doctor discontinues a therapy order based on reimbursement concerns rather than the resident's medical needs. Most commonly, a doctor discontinues therapy after receiving pressure from a Medicare contractor (an insurance company that administers Medicare reimbursement) to stop the therapy. The contractor will generally claim that the therapy is not appropriate under Medicare guidelines.

Medicare contractors also pressure nursing homes to discontinue therapy. As a result of this pressure, nursing homes become concerned that they will provide or pay for the therapy but that they will not be reimbursed by Medicare. To reduce its financial risk, a nursing home may pressure a doctor to discontinue the order for therapy, or the nursing home simply may terminate the therapy itself.

In many cases, the Medicare contractor is wrong, as discussed in detail on pages 38–41. Residents and their family members should fight for all the therapy to which the resident is entitled.

WORD TO THE WISE . . .

Enlist the help of the doctor and therapist. The residents' best allies in these disputes are often the doctor and therapist, who in many cases are just as frustrated as the resident by the pressure imposed by a Medicare contractor or other insurance company. A good strategy is to ask the doctor or therapist to make decisions based only on her medical judgment and to leave the reimbursement issues to you.

A doctor prescribing therapy can often set off a favorable chain reaction. The nursing home is required to provide the therapy, so it will work harder to justify the claim to the Medicare contractor or other insurer. The contractor or other insurer will realize that both the doctor and the nursing home are supporting the need for therapy, and it will likely authorize payment.

In pushing for therapy, however, the resident and family must consider the financial risk if the Medicare program does not ultimately cover a therapy service. Fortunately, for a resident who is also eligible for Medicaid, the financial risk is essentially nil, because a Medicaid-eligible resident cannot be charged any more than the monthly patient pay amount.

When must a nursing home make changes to meet a resident's preferences?

The Nursing Home Reform Law gives each resident the right to "reside and receive services in the facility with reasonable accommodation of individual needs and preferences, except when the health or safety of the individual or other residents would be endangered."[2] This right includes the right to make choices about his life that are significant to him and the right to choose activities, schedules, and health care.

Does a resident retain a right to privacy and confidentiality in a nursing home?

Yes. Although rooms are typically shared and space is tight, the resident has the right to privacy in all aspects of his life, including

Q & A: NURSING HOME OPERATIONS

Q. I run a nursing home, and this "reasonable accommodation" obligation seems like an impossible burden for me and my staff. How can we meet the individual needs of one hundred residents?

A. Regardless of the law, meeting your residents' needs and preferences is the right way to do business. Nothing is more destructive to a nursing home than an attitude that residents are all the same or that they are medical cases rather than human beings. Recognition of resident needs—large or small—will make residents and family members happier and will allow staff members to take real pride in the important work that they do.

Meeting individual resident needs—often called *resident-centered care*—is a cornerstone of many of the "culture change" reforms being adopted in nursing homes across the country. Two examples are the Pioneer Network (www.pioneernetwork .net) and the Eden Alternative (www.edenalt.com).

dressing, bathing, and receiving medical treatment. Staff members must close doors and curtains as needed and knock before entering closed rooms.

A resident also has the right to privacy when she receives visitors or when she communicates by telephone or mail.

Does a resident have a right to be treated with dignity?

Yes. Under a specific provision in the Nursing Home Reform Law, a resident has the right to dignity and respect from others. Nursing home staff members should be trained to be kind and courteous at all times. If a resident experiences rudeness from staff, he or his family should request that steps be taken to correct the situation.

Must a nursing home allow a resident to see the resident's medical records and receive thorough, understandable information about her care?

Yes. The Nursing Home Reform Law explicitly gives a nursing home resident the right to be fully informed about care and treatment and the right to be informed in advance about any changes in care and treatment that may affect her well-being. Information must be presented in a clear manner that is understandable to the resident. Also, a nursing home must keep thorough, accurate records for each resident and retain them for five years after the resident has left.

If a resident or resident's representative makes a request (orally or in writing) to see the resident's medical records, the nursing home must make those records available within twenty-four hours, not including weekends and holidays. The nursing home must provide copies of the medical records within two working days after receiving a request for copies. The nursing home can charge a reasonable amount for copies, based on the local price for photocopying.

**SOME DOCUMENTS THAT CAN BE
REQUESTED FROM NURSING HOME**

- Minimum data set (assessment)
- Care plan
- Doctor's orders
- Medication administration record
- Nurse's notes (regular observations of resident)
- Food intake records (including resident's weight)
- Fluid intake and output
- Incident reports
- Social worker notes

Can a nursing home provide reduced care and services to a resident who receives financial assistance from the Medicaid program?
No. The Nursing Home Reform Law protects all residents, regardless of a particular resident's form of payment. Specifically, a nursing home is not allowed to discriminate against a resident who is eligible for the Medicaid program. All residents are entitled to the same quality of service and the same staff attention regardless of how their bills are paid.[3]

This provision is one of the most important parts of the Nursing Home Reform Law but is, unfortunately, violated frequently. Discrimination against Medicaid-eligible residents is common. In the worst-offending nursing homes, the staff always is aware of who is a "Medicaid resident."

Making Choices and Planning for Care

What kinds of choices can a nursing home resident make?
Upon admission to a nursing home, a resident retains the fundamental right to control his own life. A resident does not forfeit

Q & A: SERVICES AND MEDICAID

Q. My nursing home care is covered by the Medicaid program. The nursing home tells me that the Medicaid rate is not enough, that it loses $8 a day for each Medicaid-eligible resident, and that as a result I cannot get the individual attention that I need to rehabilitate my hip. Is this right?

A. No, the nursing home is acting improperly. Remember this chapter's first rule—a nursing home is obligated to provide the services that a resident needs to attain or maintain the highest possible level of functioning.

Also, the nursing home should not be treating Medicaid-eligible residents as second-class citizens. When the nursing home applied to participate in the Medicaid program, the nursing home promised the federal and state governments that it would follow the Nursing Home Reform Law and would not discriminate against residents based on payment source. The nursing home should not break those promises—it is receiving Medicaid money only because it promised to treat Medicaid-eligible residents fairly.

If the nursing home feels that Medicaid reimbursement is inadequate, it should withdraw from the Medicaid program. It is hypocritical and improper for the nursing home to accept Medicaid money and then turn around and tell Medicaid-eligible residents that for financial reasons they will be receiving second-rate care.

rights just because he has been admitted to a nursing home. To the extent that a resident is mentally able—even if he is at times temporarily confused or forgetful—he retains the right to make basic decisions and retain control over his life.

For example, he should retain control over his general schedule, how he dresses, and how he spends his time. As is discussed on pages 107 and 128–29, the reform law requires that a nursing home make reasonable adjustments to meet a resident's preferences.

What if a resident doesn't want to undergo treatment recommended by her doctor?

A resident has the right to refuse treatment or medication, just as she would if she were living in her own home. As discussed in detail on page 149, refusal of treatment is not by itself a legitimate justification for a nursing home to evict a resident.

It is not uncommon that a resident is mentally unable to make her own health care decisions; so, her decisions are made by her representative. In general, a resident's representative has the same right as the resident to accept or refuse recommended treatment. These issues are discussed further in chapter 7.

How is a resident's nursing home care planned?

First, the nursing home staff conducts a formal assessment of the resident's condition. The assessment is used to develop a care plan. As discussed further in this chapter, the resident and family can and should participate in developing the care plan, to make sure that it reflects the resident's needs and preferences.

WORD TO THE WISE . . .

The resident is in charge. Think of the doctor and nursing home as the resident's employees. The doctor and nursing home are paid to provide the resident with expertise and health care.

The doctor and nursing home are experts, but final decisions are made by the resident or resident's representative. The resident or representative retains the right to accept or reject specific treatments.

How is an assessment performed?

The nursing home must conduct a full assessment of the resident's condition, abilities, and limitations within two weeks after the resident's admission. The assessment must be revised after significant changes in the resident's condition and reviewed at least once every three months.

The assessment must be conducted or coordinated by a registered nurse working with other nursing home staff members. The assessment must include a resident's abilities and care needs along with the resident's preferences in activities, schedules, and relationships.

Assessments are recorded in a fill-in-the-blank form called the *Minimum Data Set* or *MDS*. The MDS form is available at www.cms.hhs.gov/quality/mds20/mpaf.pdf.

After an assessment is completed, the data from the assessment form are downloaded onto a computer. These data are used to determine nursing homes' Medicare reimbursement rates and to generate the quality measures that are available on the Medicare program's Nursing Home Compare website (see pp. 22–23).

How can a resident or family member be involved in an assessment?

A resident and family should be not be shy in telling staff about the resident's needs, abilities, interests, and preferences. If the nursing home staff members are told of the resident's daily routines, religious beliefs, and favorite activities, for example, the assessment will better capture the resident as a unique individual.

What is the care plan?

The care plan describes the resident's needs and how such needs will be met, with the purpose of assisting the resident to reach or maintain the highest practicable level of functioning. The care plan must include measurable goals and timetables for meeting those goals.

A good care plan should be written in understandable language and include all of the following:

- resident's needs, including areas where assistance or improvement is needed;
- goal for each problem or need;
- approaches to achieve each goal, including who will help and how and when the planned care will be provided;
- for each goal, staff person or persons with responsibility for ensuring that the goal is accomplished; and
- timeline for evaluation and adjustment of goal and plans.

Initially, a care plan must be prepared within seven days after completion of the initial assessment. After that, a care plan must be reviewed (and revised, if necessary) at least once every three months and after any significant change in a resident's condition. Also, residents and family members can request a care plan conference whenever they believe that one is needed.

How is a care plan prepared?

A care plan is prepared by a team comprising the resident's doctor, a registered nurse from the nursing home, and other appropriate nursing home staff members. Most important, and to the extent practicable, the care plan team must include the resident, a family member or family members, and the resident's representative.

Unfortunately, the care-planning process is sometimes treated by a nursing home or family as an unimportant formality. For example, a nursing home may write the same vague care plan for virtually all of its residents. Or a resident's family member may skip the care plan meetings scheduled by the nursing home.

This attitude—whether held by the nursing home or the resident's family—can lead to dramatically poor care for the resident. If the resident's care plan becomes a meaningless piece of paper,

---

WORD TO THE WISE . . .

Don't settle for second-class care. If nursing home staff members are accustomed to just going through the motions in the development of a care plan, a resident or family member will have to take the initiative. What does the resident need or want? Ask for it!

And don't feel apologetic or guilty for asking that the resident, for example, be taken around the block in her wheelchair each day or that she be allowed to get out of bed relatively late in the morning. The nursing home is paid thousands of dollars each month to care for the resident and is required by the Nursing Home Reform Law to satisfy resident preferences to the extent possible.

Further information about care planning is available in the book *Nursing Homes: Getting Good Care There*, available from the National Citizens' Coalition for Nursing Home Reform at (202) 332-2275 and www.nccnhr.org.

---

then the resident may receive nothing more than meals and supervision. It is important that a resident and his family work with the nursing home to have a strong care plan, individualized to reflect the resident's needs and preferences.

How is a doctor involved in a resident's care?

A nursing home must ensure that each resident's care is supervised by a doctor selected by the resident or the resident's representative. The nursing home must also ensure that an alternate doctor is available, in case of an emergency.

WORD TO THE WISE . . .

Finding a doctor may be difficult. The resident has the right to choose his own doctor. However, as a practical matter, many doctors refuse to visit patients in nursing homes. A resident should check with his doctor and with the nursing home to find out which doctors are willing to come to the nursing home to see patients.

Because many doctors are unwilling to visit nursing homes, a doctor who is willing to visit a nursing home often becomes the doctor of record for many residents. Often, but not always, this doctor also serves as the nursing home's medical director.

It can be a good or bad sign that a doctor follows a high percentage of a nursing home's residents. The best-case scenario is that the doctor takes a special interest in nursing home care. The worst-case scenario is that the doctor is not particularly successful and has turned to nursing home care because a nursing home can provide him with a large number of patients.

The unfortunate bottom line for residents is that the right to choose a doctor may not be as powerful is it might initially seem, because many doctors are not willing to make the required monthly visit to a nursing home resident.

The resident's doctor must generally visit and evaluate the resident when medically appropriate and at least once every thirty days.

The nursing home must keep the resident's doctor informed of a resident's condition. For example, the nursing home must notify the doctor of a sudden or marked change in a resident's condition or a significant change in weight.

General Care

What must a nursing home do to ensure that a resident's simple, daily needs are met?

Under the Nursing Home Reform Law, a nursing home is expected to help a resident to maintain or improve her ability to bathe, dress, groom, walk, eat, talk, and use the toilet. These activities are called "activities of daily living." The law specifically states that a nursing home "must ensure that [a] resident's abilities in the activities of daily living do not diminish unless circumstances of the individual's clinical condition demonstrate that diminution was unavoidable."[4]

If a resident is unable to perform any of the activities of daily living, the nursing home is required to assist the resident accordingly. A resident requiring help in eating must be provided with assistance or, if appropriate, with special equipment to enable independent eating.

In providing assistance, a nursing home must help a resident remain as independent as possible, even if it is easier for the staff to simply take over a task for a resident. Assume, for example, that a resident can feed herself if she is helped by a nurse aide but that the nursing home could save time and money by having the nursing aide feed the resident or by having a feeding tube inserted into the resident. In this situation, the nursing home must direct the nurse aide to help the resident feed herself. By doing so, the nursing home maintains the resident's independence as much as is possible.

What must a nursing home do to maintain a resident's ability to move his limbs?

Under the reform law, a resident without limitations in how he moves should "not experience reduction in range of motion unless the resident's clinical condition demonstrates that a reduction in range of motion is unavoidable." A resident with a limited range of motion must receive "appropriate treatment and services to increase range of motion and/or to prevent further decrease in range of motion."[5] Physical restraints are not to be applied unless unavoidable; restraints are discussed in detail on pages 124–28.

What rehabilitation services must a nursing home provide?

Consistent with the aforementioned requirements, the reform law requires that a nursing home provide rehabilitation services for the improvement or maintenance of a resident's condition. These rehabilitation services include, but are not limited to, physical therapy,

---

WORD TO THE WISE . . .

Push for therapy under Medicare or Medicaid. Be alert if a resident has received therapy under Medicare nursing home coverage and the Medicare coverage now is ending. Check with the doctor to make sure that the doctor's continuing recommendations regarding therapy are based on medical considerations, not reimbursement calculations. If a nursing home on its own discontinues prescribed therapy, politely and professionally inform the nursing home that the reform law requires that prescribed therapy be provided regardless of the reimbursement source.

A Medicaid-eligible resident cannot be charged any more than the monthly Medicaid patient pay amount for nursing home care, regardless of the therapy services provided. Of course, a resident paying privately can be liable for additional therapy services, if the nursing home admission agreement sets out an additional charge for therapy services and the therapy is not covered by Medicare or other type of insurance program.

Payment for therapy by Medicare Part A is discussed in detail on pages 38–42.

> ## Q & A: MEDICAID AND THERAPY
>
> **Q.** My nursing home tells me that I cannot get physical therapy because my payments are made by the Medicaid program. Can the nursing home refuse to give me therapy that the doctor has prescribed?
>
> **A.** No. The reform law requires that a nursing home provide all residents with prescribed therapy. This law applies no matter how a resident's nursing home bill is paid.[6]

occupational therapy, and speech therapy, as prescribed by a doctor's order. Significantly, a rehabilitation service must be provided to any resident for whom the service has been prescribed, including a Medicaid-eligible resident. This is so even if the nursing home is reimbursed at the same Medicaid rate whether therapy is provided or not.

What activities must a nursing home provide for its residents?

A nursing home must provide activities for its residents. An activity program must follow a written, planned schedule.

Good activities are designed to engage and interest residents. A nursing home should have different types of activities for different types of residents. An activity may be appropriate for a mentally alert resident, for example, but completely inappropriate for a resident with significant dementia. Activities should respect and incorporate a resident's cultural and religious background.

Medical Conditions

What must a nursing home do to prevent or treat pressure sores?

Again, the general rule is that a nursing home must prevent a resident's decline as much as possible. A resident without pressure

WORD TO THE WISE . . .

Think creatively to plan activities. In too many nursing homes, the activity program is principally a large television that runs from morning to night. Residents deserve better. Again, think creatively. What would the resident enjoy?

This is another instance when a nursing home can benefit from energy and ideas brought by a resident and family. A functioning activities program can make day-to-day life more pleasurable for residents and staff members alike.

sores (also known as *bed sores*, *pressure ulcers*, or *decubitus ulcers*) should not develop them "unless the [resident's] clinical condition demonstrates that they were unavoidable."[7]

Pressure sores develop when pressure on an area of the body shuts down blood vessels and deprives that body area of oxygen and nutrients. Pressure sores can be prevented by keeping pressure off at-risk areas of the body, keeping skin clean, and maintaining good nutrition. At-risk areas include the buttocks, heels, and coccyx (tailbone).

To relieve pressure on residents' skin, a nursing home must turn or shift residents who would otherwise be immobile in a bed or wheelchair. Clinical guidelines developed by the federal government recommend that a bed-bound resident be turned at least every two hours and that a resident in a wheelchair be shifted at least hourly.

If a resident develops pressure sores, a nursing home must provide the treatment necessary to heal the sores and prevent infection. A nursing home must notify the resident's doctor when a pressure sore develops and when treatment of such a sore has not been effective.

WORD TO THE WISE . . .

Examine pressure sore statistics. Statistics on the pressure sore frequency at an individual nursing home can be found at the Medicare program's Nursing Home Compare website. Go to www.medicare.gov and select the search tool "Compare Nursing Homes in Your Area." More information on Nursing Home Compare is available on pages 22–23.

How must a nursing home help a resident control his urine?

A resident without adequate control of his bladder must receive treatment to restore normal bladder functioning as much as possible. Specifically, if a resident needs assistance to go to the bathroom frequently or to use a toilet or bedpan, then the nursing home must provide that assistance. A resident should not be given a catheter or diaper unless it is a medical necessity, even if the nursing home could save time and money by using one or the other.

If a resident does have a catheter, the nursing home must monitor the resident's fluid intake and output. The nursing home must provide treatment to prevent and, if necessary, treat urinary tract infections.

Is specialized care available for terminally ill residents?

Yes, this specialized care is known as *hospice care*. Hospice services in a nursing home are generally paid by the Medicare program and provided by an outside hospice agency that supplements the nursing home's care.

Hospice care is a method of caring for the terminally ill that emphasizes supportive services rather than cure. Hospice care generally involves a team approach of doctors, nurses, social workers, clergy, counselors, and therapists, depending on individual and family needs.

Hospice care is available under Medicare Part A if all of the following conditions are met: the patient is eligible for Medicare Part A coverage; the patient's doctor and the hospice medical director certify that the patient likely has six months or less to live; the patient signs a statement choosing hospice care instead of standard Medicare benefits for the terminal illness; and the patient receives care from a Medicare-approved hospice program.

A Medicare beneficiary is entitled to two ninety-day periods of hospice care, a subsequent thirty-day period, and then a potentially unlimited number of sixty-day periods. For each period, a doctor must certify that the patient is terminally ill.

The Medicare program publishes a helpful guide entitled *Medicare Hospice Benefits*. The guide is available by calling 1-800-MEDICARE and by accessing the Internet at www.medicare.gov/Publications/Pubs/pdf/02154_LE.pdf.

WORD TO THE WISE . . .

Consider hospice care. The hospice benefit is tremendously underused. Most Medicare beneficiaries die without using it. Even those who use the benefit often start hospice care only a week or two before death.

Hospice services can be a comforting presence for both a terminally ill resident and her family. This guide encourages terminally ill residents and their families to talk honestly about the resident's prognosis and to consider seriously the possibility of using hospice services.

This advice, of course, falls into the easier-said-than-done category. Talking about impending death is not easy. But dealing with impending death is not easy either, and the assistance of a hospice agency can ease the burden for everyone involved.

Access to Medical Services and Medications

How does a nursing home provide medications?

Under the reform law, a nursing home must ensure that residents receive prescribed medications. Because many nursing home residents are Medicare beneficiaries, much medication is obtained through Medicare Part D prescription drug coverage. Each Part D plan is required to have long-term care pharmacies in the plan's networks, and these pharmacies must provide medications in any special packaging needed by nursing homes.

More information about Medicare Part D is available on pages 47–49.

Is a nursing home required to provide mental health services?

Consistent with the principle that a nursing home must help each resident achieve the highest possible level of functioning, a nursing home must provide or arrange for appropriate mental health services if an assessment indicates that the resident has problems in adjusting to his environment.

On a practical level, most nursing homes do not recognize mental health issues except when those issues manifest themselves

---

WORD TO THE WISE . . .

Don't assume that depression is normal. Depression and other mental illness should not be considered normal or unavoidable. Family members should pay attention to whether the resident is avoiding social interaction or showing signs of depression or other mental illness. If the resident appears to be suffering from a mental illness, the family should request that the nursing home conduct an assessment and obtain appropriate services.

as "behavioral problems." Nursing homes typically respond by attempting to control or restrain the resident. Depression and anxiety are often ignored when they should be treated with standard mental health measures, such as crisis intervention services, psychotherapy, and drug therapy.

Must a nursing home provide access to dental care, vision care, and other special services?

A nursing home must arrange for its residents to receive necessary dental, vision, hearing, and foot care, although the nursing home is not required to pay for such services. Services must be provided on-site, or transportation to outside care must be available.

Nursing homes are required to ensure that residents have access to a variety of special services, including respiratory care, foot care, and care for a prosthesis, although again, the nursing home is not required to provide such services directly or pay for them.

Minimizing Use of Physical and Chemical Restraints

What is a physical restraint?

Federal guidelines define physical restraints broadly, stating that any device or material that "restricts freedom of movement or normal access to [a resident's] body" is a physical restraint.[8] "Leg restraints, arm restraints, hand mitts, soft ties, vest[s], wheelchair safety bars, and geri-chairs are physical restraints." A bed rail or a lap tray can also be a physical restraint. Even a chair angled in such a way to prevent the resident from rising or a tight tucking into bed can be a physical restraint.

When can a resident be restrained?

Under the Nursing Home Reform Law, a nursing home resident "has the right to be free from any physical . . . restraints imposed

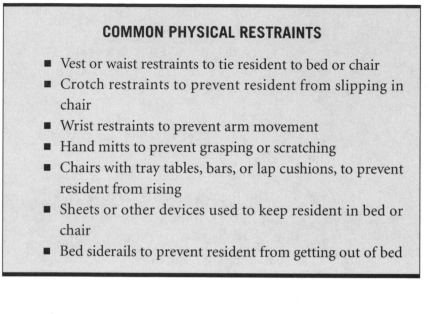

COMMON PHYSICAL RESTRAINTS

- Vest or waist restraints to tie resident to bed or chair
- Crotch restraints to prevent resident from slipping in chair
- Wrist restraints to prevent arm movement
- Hand mitts to prevent grasping or scratching
- Chairs with tray tables, bars, or lap cushions, to prevent resident from rising
- Sheets or other devices used to keep resident in bed or chair
- Bed siderails to prevent resident from getting out of bed

for purposes of discipline or convenience, and not required to treat the resident's medical symptoms." Except for emergency situations, "restraints may only be imposed to ensure the physical safety of the resident or other residents and only upon the written order of a physician that specifies the duration and circumstances under which the restraints are to be used."

In summary, physical restraints cannot be used for discipline or the nursing home's convenience. Restraints require a doctor's order.

Who decides if and when physical restraints should be used?

A restraint is a medical procedure and must be ordered by a resident's doctor. Like any doctor's order in a nursing home, an order for restraints cannot be implemented without the consent of the resident or the resident's representative.

A resident or resident's representative should demand the right to determine the use of restraints on the resident. A resident or resident's representative should feel free to refuse undesired restraints,

---

Q & A: SIDERAILS

Q. The nursing home wants to put siderails on my mother's bed to prevent her from leaving the bed at night and possibly falling. The director of nursing says that it will be easier for the nursing home if siderails are used. Does my mother have to accept siderails?

A. No. A siderail is a physical restraint when used to prevent a resident from getting out of bed, and the use of siderails is being proposed for the nursing home's convenience. Your mother can and should refuse their use.

Consider alternatives to siderails. A better alternative may be a bed that can be lowered to just a foot or two from the floor, along with the placement of cushions next to the bed.

---

even if this choice contradicts the doctor's orders or the nursing home's preferences.

Can a nursing home insist on applying restraints unless and until a resident or resident's representative releases the nursing home from legal responsibility for the resident's health and safety?

No. A nursing home cannot avoid its legal obligations to provide adequate care and supervision.

The nursing home can require that a resident or resident's representative make a written decision to request or refuse physical restraints. Any such written decision, however, cannot limit the nursing home's legal responsibility.

Can a nursing home medicate a resident to make him "manageable"?

Under the reform law, a behavior-modifying medication—also called a *psychoactive medication* and sometimes a *chemical restraint*—can

WORD TO THE WISE . . .

Think carefully about restraints. The use of physical restraints has dropped drastically over the past fifteen years, and many facilities now function completely restraint-free. Part of this decline is certainly due to the reform law's restriction on the use of physical restraints.

Another part of the decline is due to a growing medical consensus that, instead of protecting residents, restraints harm residents, both physically and psychologically. By limiting a resident's ability to move, restraints may cause a resident to become even more unsteady and susceptible to falls and injuries.

That being said, physical restraints remain an option. The ultimate decision on the use of restraints rests with the resident or, more likely, the resident's representative and depends on the facts of the particular situation. In making the decision, the resident or resident's representative should make sure that the use of restraints is a last resort and should be aware of the considerable research on how the use of physical restraints can be limited or virtually eliminated. See, for example, the "Untie the Elderly" resources at www.ute.kendal.org, assembled by the nonprofit Kendal Corporation.

If and when restraints are recommended, a resident's representative may want to discuss the issues in a care plan meeting. The care-planning process is a good opportunity to discuss the pros and cons of restraints and to examine possible alternatives.

WORD TO THE WISE . . .

Consider whether behavior-modifying medication is being recommended for the resident's good or the nursing home's convenience. Note that behavior-modifying medications can and should be used as appropriate to treat various psychological and emotional conditions—schizophrenia, paranoia, or depression, for example. In deciding whether use of a particular medication is advisable, a good rule of thumb is to consider whether the medication is intended for the resident's benefit to treat a specifically diagnosed health problem or is meant for the nursing home's benefit to keep the resident manageable.

If the benefit is to the resident, then use of the medication is likely advisable. If, on the other hand, use of the medication would be primarily for the nursing home's benefit—for example, to keep the resident quiet and out of the way—then the medication should likely be refused.

The most important point with behavior-modifying medications is the right of the resident or, more likely, the resident's representative to decide whether to use them. If a resident's representative thinks that the use of such medication would be unwise, premature, or excessive, he should feel free to say no.

A care-planning meeting is a good forum in which to discuss issues relating to medication. A resident's representative should not be coerced into approving a behavior-modifying medication that does not benefit the resident. If the use of such medication is recommended by the doctor or nursing home staff members, the representative should ask the doctor or staff members to propose alternatives.

be used only to treat a resident's medical conditions or symptoms. Behavior-modifying medication cannot be used for discipline or the nursing home's convenience.

Like any other medication, behavior-modifying medication can be administered only with the consent of the resident or—if the resident does not have mental capacity to consent—the resident's representative. If behavior-modifying medication is recommended by the resident's doctor, the resident or resident's representative must be told what condition or illness is being treated and then have the choice whether to accept or reject the recommendation.

Meals and Schedules

How must a nursing home serve meals and snacks?
A nursing home must provide residents with at least three meals each day. Dinner during the evening and breakfast the following morning cannot be separated by more than fourteen hours. Snacks must be available at bedtime. To prevent dehydration, drinks should be available at all times.

A nursing home is required to address a resident's specific nutritional needs as well as follow doctor-ordered diets. A nursing home is required to make "reasonable accommodations" for a resident's preferences, making substitutions from appropriate food

---

WORD TO THE WISE . . .

Seek meal choices. As discussed, a nursing home must offer choices in the food served. A well-run nursing home will recognize meal choices as an opportunity to build goodwill. By offering a choice of food, a nursing home can reduce complaints and give itself an attractive selling point.

groups. Ideally, a facility would offer ethnic meals that are appropriate for residents' cultural backgrounds.

More information on a nursing home's obligation to meet resident preferences is available on page 107.

Is a resident obligated to follow the same schedule as that of every other resident?

No. When organizing residents' schedules, a nursing home must make reasonable accommodations to meet residents' individual needs and preferences. For example, if a resident prefers to sleep until 8:00 AM, the nursing home should not wake the resident at 6:30 AM. The nursing home can comply with the law by waking the resident at 8:00 AM and by having cereal, fruit, and juice available for residents who get up after the standard breakfast time.

Staffing Requirements

If a nursing home does not have enough staff members to provide required services, is the nursing home excused from the laws discussed in this chapter?

No. In many instances, a nursing home will claim that it does not have enough staff members to provide the individualized care required by law. When confronted with this argument, a resident

---

WORD TO THE WISE . . .

Staffing information is on the Internet. Information on a nursing home's staffing levels can be found on the Medicare program's Nursing Home Compare website. Go to www.medicare.gov and select the search tool "Compare Nursing Homes in Your Area." More information on Nursing Home Compare is available on pages 22–23.

or family member should insist that the nursing home comply with legal requirements and, if necessary, hire additional staff members.

Notes

1. This regulation is found at section 483.25 of Title 42 of the Code of Federal Regulations.

2. This regulation is found at section 483.15(e)(1) of Title 42 of the Code of Federal Regulations.

3. This regulation is found at section 483.12(c)(1) of Title 42 of the Code of Federal Regulations.

4. This regulation is found at section 483.25(a)(1) of Title 42 of the Code of Federal Regulations.

5. The range-of-motion regulations are found at section 483.25(e) of Title 42 of the Code of Federal Regulations.

6. The relevant language is as follows: "Specialized rehabilitative services are considered facility services and are, thus, included within the scope of facility services. They must be provided to residents who need them even when the services are not specifically enumerated in the State [Medicaid] plan. No fee can be charged a Medicaid recipient for specialized rehabilitative services because they are covered facility services." This language is found in the Surveyor's Guidelines to section 483.45(a) of Title 42 of the Code of Federal Regulations. These guidelines are contained in appendix PP to the *State Operations Manual of the Centers for Medicare and Medicaid Services.*

7. This regulation is found at section 483.25(c) of Title 42 of the Code of Federal Regulations.

8. This regulation is found at section 483.13(a) of Title 42 of the Code of Federal Regulations.

Residents' Health Care Decision Making

- Introduction
- General Principles
- Appointing an Agent
- When No Agent Is Appointed
- Nursing Homes
- Right to Die

Introduction

Nursing home residents have the right to make their own health care decisions as long as they are of sound mind. If, however, they are incapacitated or unable to communicate—for example, because of a stroke, coma, disease, or accident—their health care choices are best followed when a legal representative authorizes the health care or when the resident had given adequate instructions in a legally recognized way.

The message: Planning ahead is the best way to ensure that a resident's wishes are known and followed.

This chapter reviews health care decision making generally and then addresses appointment of an agent. It discusses what happens when no agent is appointed, as well as nursing home responsibilities and right-to-die issues.

General Principles

What written documents can be used to specify preferences regarding future health care?

In every state, an individual can prepare a document to specify preferences regarding future health care. The specific documents vary somewhat from state to state. Most documents fall into one of the following two categories:

> *Power of Attorney for Health Care*, also known as a *proxy*. An individual appoints another person—known as the *agent*, *attorney-in-fact*, or *proxy*—to make health care decisions for the individual in the future. In addition, the individual can generally list instructions regarding future health

---

Q & A: USING FORMS

Q. Is it really necessary to search out the correct form? I'm going to save time and money by using a Living Will form that I found in a magazine.

A. Why would you put yourself—and your family and friends—at risk for the sake of a few dollars and a few hours? Don't rely on magazine forms, informal written statements, or the "Documentation of Preferred Intensity of Care" papers used by many nursing homes. These documents are not recognized by state law.

care. This document can be broad and flexible to cover many situations.

Health Care Directive, also called a *living will.* An individual can list instructions regarding future health care. Medical professionals must generally follow these instructions. This document is limited—it usually applies only to end-of-life decisions.

Which is better: a Power of Attorney for Health Care or a Health Care Directive?

A Power of Attorney for Health Care is generally more effective because an agent can be given authority over all of the resident's health care decisions. A Health Care Directive, on the other hand, is effective only for those health care situations specifically discussed in the directive.

In some states, the answer to the "Which is better?" question is "both." In these states, an individual uses a Power of Attorney for Health Care to appoint an agent and uses the Health Care Directive to list preferences regarding specific health care decisions.

A Health Care Directive is particularly useful for those residents who have no family member or friend who is able or willing to act as an agent. In that case, a Health Care Directive may be a resident's only option.

WORD TO THE WISE . . .

Find the correct form. Health care decision-making documents have differing names and formats in different states. Since state law applies, it is important to use the format recognized in the state where the resident resides. The specific advance directives used in each state are available online from the National Hospice and Palliative Care Organization, at www.caringinfo.org.

Does a resident need to hire an attorney to create a Power of Attorney for Health Care or a Health Care Directive?

No, not necessarily. Although attorneys prepare both Powers of Attorney for Health Care and Health Care Directives, either document often can be completed with a relatively inexpensive fill-in-the-blanks form. If a resident's desires are relatively straightforward, a form document is generally adequate. The form must follow the law of the state in which the resident is residing at the time the form is completed.

A mentally competent resident generally can complete a form simply by following the directions on the form. Requirements for signing and witnessing vary from state to state. The signature of a notary public may or may not be required.

Regardless, it is best if an attorney coordinates all of a resident's planning—the documents relating to health care decision making, along with documents relating to financial decision making and the post-death handling of the resident's affairs.

How should a resident notify others that she has appointed an agent through a Power of Attorney for Health Care or signed a Health Care Directive?

A resident should give copies of the document to family members, to the nursing home, and to her doctor and hospital. The original documents should be kept where an agent can find them.

WORD TO THE WISE . . .

Make copies. Copies are cheap. Make multiple copies of your health care documents and distribute them to family, friends, doctors, hospitals, HMOs, and other health care personnel and facilities.

If a resident has appointed an agent through a Power of Attorney for Health Care, the resident should prepare a card that lists the telephone number of the resident's agent and then keep the card in her wallet.

How long will a Power of Attorney for Health Care or a Health Care Directive remain effective?

Once completed, a Power of Attorney for Health Care or a Health Care Directive generally remains effective indefinitely, unless the document specifies an expiration date. While the individual is of sound mind, he may revoke or revise either document at any time. It is a good idea to review a Power of Attorney for Health Care or Health Care Directive every couple of years and make revisions as necessary.

WORD TO THE WISE . . .

Redo the forms after moving to another state. If possible, redo documents when you move to another state. Although health care providers are, in general, legally obligated to accept documents that were prepared in other states, they are more often comfortable with their respective state documents.

Appointing an Agent

Why should a resident appoint another person to make health care decisions for her?

Many nursing home residents are of sound mind. Any resident, however, may become incapacitated in the future. In addition, surgical procedures and other medical treatments may create situations in which a resident is temporarily unable to make health care decisions. Consequently, a resident should prepare now to ensure that she receives appropriate health care if she ever becomes incapacitated or is temporarily unable to communicate.

If a resident has no legal representative when she becomes incapacitated, she may not be able to receive needed medical treatment. Also, an incapacitated resident without a legal representative may not be able to refuse medical treatment that will only prolong the resident's pain, even if she has no real prospect of recovery.

On the other hand, if a person has been appointed to make health care decisions for an incapacitated resident, those decisions can be made in a way most consistent with the resident's expressed desires.

The previous discussion applies to everyone, not just to nursing home residents. Persons of all ages and health conditions can benefit by appointing a family member or friend to make health care decisions if and when the appointing person becomes incapacitated.

WORD TO THE WISE . . .

Every adult should do it. Every adult—whether in a nursing home or not—should select a health care agent and complete a Power of Attorney for Health Care and, when appropriate, a Health Care Directive.

How can a resident appoint another person to make health care decisions for the resident?

A legally competent adult can create a Power of Attorney for Health Care or similar document. The Power of Attorney for Health Care is a legally binding document that allows the person appointed (the "agent") to make sure that the resident's health care instructions are followed. The Power of Attorney for Health Care thus allows a doctor, hospital, or nursing home to receive clear instructions even if the resident no longer can make health care decisions. In many states, the agent can be given broad authority to make all decisions about medical care.

The Power of Attorney for Health Care usually is drafted to take effect when the resident becomes incapacitated and only for the duration of the incapacity. For example, if a resident undergoes surgery and recovers, the authority of the agent to make health care decisions for the resident under the Power of Attorney expires when the resident is again able to communicate.

Whom should a resident select as his agent under a Power of Attorney for Health Care?

The agent can be a family member, friend, or other person. A resident probably should select a person who knows him well, can follow his wishes, and can discuss life-and-death issues with him. Ideally, the agent will be someone who can be physically present when decisions have to be made, although out of necessity an agent is sometimes an out-of-state adult child.

Personality matters. Ideally, the agent will be congenial enough to have polite conversations with health care providers and family members but also strong enough to not be coerced or intimidated when a difficult decision has to be made.

The agent should generally not be a health care provider to the resident or an owner or employee of the nursing home, unless also a relative of the resident. Laws vary from state to state about who cannot be the agent.

The resident should always select one or two alternate agents in case the primary agent is unable or unwilling to act. Naming two persons together as co-agents is usually not a good idea, because of the possibility that they may find themselves in an irreconcilable disagreement.

Can a resident give specific instructions to an agent appointed through a Power of Attorney for Health Care?

Yes, generally. Also, depending on the state, a Power of Attorney for Health Care form may provide an optional section in which a resident can declare her desire to receive or not receive life-sustaining treatment under certain conditions. These optional sections also often provide space for a resident to list any instructions relating to health care decisions that she wishes to express.

WORD TO THE WISE . . .

Discuss preferences and beliefs with family and friends. A resident should discuss personal preferences and beliefs with his health care agent and put these preferences in writing wherever possible. In addition to making written instructions, a resident should discuss his preferences with the agent. Discussing health care decisions while the resident is able to explain his desires can give the agent a sense of comfort about difficult decisions that may have to be made in the future.

What kinds of health care decisions can an agent make for an incapacitated resident?

In most states, a broadly written Power of Attorney for Health Care allows an agent to make any and all health care and treatment decisions for an incapacitated resident, subject to the resident's instructions listed in the Power of Attorney for Health Care or Health Care Directive. For example, the agent can potentially do all of the following:

- Consent to or refuse any medical treatment
- Authorize, withhold, or withdraw life-sustaining procedures

HELPFUL RESOURCES

■ *Your Way*, a guide to discussing and choosing future health care, is available from the Healthcare and Elder Law Programs Corporation (HELP) of Torrance, California; 310-533-1996; www.help4srs.org.

■ The *Consumer's Tool Kit for Advance Health Care Planning* contains worksheets to assist persons to clarify and communicate their wishes. The kit is available from the American Bar Association, 202-662-8690; www.abanet.org/aging/toolkit/home.html.

■ Hire or fire medical providers and authorize admission to medical facilities, including nursing homes
■ Review medical records

When No Agent Is Appointed

Can a resident give instructions about future health care without appointing an agent?

Yes. In most states, a Health Care Directive enables an individual to state her desires about future health care. These instructions must be honored by future health care providers, if at a later time the individual is no longer capable of making her own health care decisions.

To give adequate direction to those health care providers, the individual should list her instructions as specifically as possible.

Can a family member or friend make health care decisions for an incapacitated or unable-to-communicate resident if the resident never appointed an agent?

Yes, generally, although the law varies quite a bit from state to state.

As a practical matter, the nearest relative of an incapacitated or unable-to-communicate resident generally makes health care decisions for the resident if no one else has been appointed to make those decisions. In some states, this practice is supported by a preference order established by state law. For example, state law may specify that the spouse of an incapacitated individual has authority to make the individual's health care decisions. If there is no spouse, state law might appoint a child; if there is no spouse and no child, state law might appoint a parent or a sibling.

Not all states' laws have preference orders. In these states, a health care provider is likely to take instructions from the nearest relative, in part because it seems like the right thing to do and in part because there is some support for this practice in court decisions.

Although, as discussed, the nearest relative is often recognized as the appropriate decision maker, this informal recognition is sometimes not enough. Perhaps the "wrong" person is given authority—for example, if the individual was estranged from his spouse but the law nonetheless gives her authority over his health care decisions. Or perhaps the incapacitated individual has three children, and they can't agree on what should be done.

Also, even if the "right" person is given authority under state law, the nursing home or other health care provider may be hesitant to recognize this authority. The nursing home or health care provider may be more comfortable accepting health care decisions from an agent appointed under a Power of Attorney for Health Care or from a family member or friend who has been appointed by a court.

The relevant court procedure is called a *conservatorship* in some states and an *adult guardianship* in others. In either procedure, a court appoints someone to act indefinitely on behalf of an incapacitated adult. The person appointed (the "conservator" or "guardian") can be given the power to determine the medical treatment, residence, and/or finances of the incapacitated adult (the "conservatee" or "ward").

A family member or friend desiring a conservatorship/ guardianship should consult with a knowledgeable attorney. The resident has the right to be present in court with her own attorney and to consent or object.

WORD TO THE WISE . . .

An ounce of prevention is worth a pound of cure. A conservatorship or guardianship can be expensive and complicated. It is better for a resident, when mentally competent, to create a Power of Attorney for Health Care or a Health Care Directive.

Who makes health care decisions for an incapacitated resident who did not appoint an agent and who has no family members or friends willing to act as a legal representative?

The answer to this question varies from state to state and from situation to situation. If the resident has some financial resources, a professional conservator or guardian may apply to be appointed conservator/guardian and to receive payment from the resident's money. In some states, a local government agency such as a public guardian will apply to be appointed conservator/guardian.

Nursing Homes

Can a nursing home require a resident to sign a Power of Attorney for Health Care or Health Care Directive?

No. The Nursing Home Reform Law prohibits a nursing home from conditioning admission or continued stay on a resident's possession (or nonpossession) of a Power of Attorney for Health Care,

Health Care Directive, or any other advance directive for health care.

In addition, the reform law requires that a nursing home inform an incoming resident of her right to accept or refuse medical treatment and her ability to create a Power of Attorney for Health Care or Health Care Directive. If the resident chooses to create any type of advance directive, the nursing home must document that choice in the resident's medical record.

Must a nursing home obey the decisions of an agent appointed under a Power of Attorney for Health Care or the instructions of a Health Care Directive?

In general, yes, although state law may provide for some limited exceptions. In many states, a nursing home is not required to follow a decision or instruction if the nursing home objects to it as a matter of conscience. For example, a nursing home affiliated with a religious denomination may refuse to withhold life-sustaining treatment from a terminally ill resident based on the nursing home's religious principles. Residents must be informed of any such conscience-based policy at the time of admission—otherwise, the nursing home cannot use that policy against the resident.

WORD TO THE WISE . . .

Conscience-based policies are rare. A nursing home almost never has a conscience-based policy that allows it to ignore the decision of a resident or agent. Virtually the only exception is the situation discussed in the text—a religion-affiliated nursing home with a policy against the withholding or withdrawal of life-sustaining treatment.

Under most state laws, a nursing home is obligated to accept an out-of-state Power of Attorney for Health Care or a Health Care Directive if the resident was living in that state when the document was signed.

Right to Die

Can a resident choose to make health care decisions that likely will hasten the resident's death?

Yes, a right to refuse treatment is established by the U.S. Constitution and, for nursing home residents, the Nursing Home Reform Law. As discussed on page 149, a resident's refusal of treatment, by itself, almost never justifies eviction from the nursing home.

Can a resident specify that she be allowed to die under certain circumstances?

Yes, probably. As discussed earlier in this chapter, a resident can sign a Power of Attorney for Health Care and/or Health Care Directive to (1) appoint an agent to make health care decisions for the resident if the resident loses the ability to make such decisions and/or (2) specify the conditions under which the resident would not wish to receive life-sustaining treatment.

In some states, decisions to refuse life-sustaining treatment must meet relatively strict requirements to be honored.

Will a paramedic attempt to resuscitate a dying resident although that resident has requested through a legal document that he be allowed to die?

Quite probably. During an emergency call, most paramedics don't have the time to read Powers of Attorney for Health Care or Health Care Directives.

Of course, if a resident or a resident's agent has legally chosen to refuse life-sustaining treatment, the nursing home should not call

911 in the first place. In many cases, however, nursing home staff will call 911 even for residents who have declined life-sustaining treatment because the staff has overlooked the resident's request or does not want to take the responsibility of withholding life-sustaining treatment.

To ensure that a paramedic will be aware of a decision to refuse life-sustaining treatment, a resident should wear a do-not-resuscitate bracelet or medallion, available from the MedicAlert Foundation at (888) 633-4298 or www.medicalert.org.

Can an incapacitated resident be allowed to die if she, while still competent, did not execute a legal request for limited medical treatment?
Maybe. The law on this question differs from state to state. Consult a knowledgeable attorney on this issue.

8

Staying in the Nursing Home

- Introduction
- Eviction Overview
- Eviction Procedures
- Readmission after Absences from the Nursing Home: Bed-Hold Rules
- Transfers within a Nursing Home

Introduction

After getting into a nursing home and becoming familiar with it, a resident and family may believe that the resident is well settled. They will be shocked if the nursing home later decides to move the resident. A nursing home may threaten a move for a variety of reasons, many of which are illegal.

This chapter first provides an overview of eviction rules. Then it reviews eviction procedures and discusses readmission after absences. Finally, it presents information on transfers within a nursing home.

Eviction Overview

When can a nursing home evict a resident?

Nursing home residents, like tenants in an apartment building, generally have the right to stay where they are living. If the nursing home accepts Medicare or Medicaid funds (and thus must obey the federal Nursing Home Reform Law), a resident can be evicted only under one of five circumstances:

1. The nursing home cannot meet the resident's needs, and as a result the resident's welfare requires evicting the resident.
2. The health of the resident has improved so that he no longer needs the services of a nursing home.
3. The resident's presence in the nursing home endangers the health or safety of others in the nursing home.
4. The resident has failed to pay for her stay at the nursing home, despite having received reasonable and appropriate notice of nonpayment.
5. The nursing home is ceasing operations.

Other than for these five reasons, a nursing home generally is not allowed to evict a resident. As much as possible, a nursing home should feel like a resident's home, not like a short-stay hospital. For that reason, the reform law protects a resident's right to remain in a nursing home, even if the resident's continued stay might be considered inconvenient or costly for the nursing home.

WORD TO THE WISE . . .

Beware of improper reasons. Nursing homes claim many improper reasons for eviction. This chapter discusses many commonly claimed but improper reasons.

Improper Reason: Time-Consuming Care Needs

"Care for you has become too difficult and time-consuming. We can no longer meet your needs, so we're transferring you down the street to Shady Tree Convalescent Hospital."

Why the nursing home is wrong. The resident does not need a higher level of care, such as that of a hospital or an acute psychiatric facility. He needs nursing home care, as shown by the fact that the nursing home intends to transfer him to another nursing home—Shady Tree Convalescent Hospital.

As discussed in detail in chapter 6, a nursing home is obligated to make available an array of services. The fact is that the nursing home is generally obligated by law to provide the level of care that the resident requires. The rare exceptions are generally situations when the resident needs particular specialized equipment—for example, when the resident needs to be on a ventilator.

Improper Reason: Difficult Behavior

"Your mother has aggressive dementia and is cantankerous and obnoxious. All she does is criticize, which is why ten aides have asked to be transferred to another wing of the nursing home. We're transferring your mother to another nursing home."

Why the nursing home is wrong. The resident is evidently not a danger to the safety or health of other residents. Nursing home care is the right kind of care for her, as shown by the fact that the nursing home intends to transfer her to another nursing home.

Nursing homes often attempt to evict residents with dementia who have unpleasant or difficult behaviors. In almost all such occasions, the nursing home is wrong. A nursing home is likely the right place for an individual with aggressive dementia, and nursing homes are obligated by the reform law and medical standards to provide comprehensive dementia care.

Nothing is gained by nursing homes' attempting to dump their difficult residents on other nursing homes. When a resident with dementia exhibits difficult behavior, the nursing home should respond not by attempting to transfer the resident but by returning to the care-planning process to determine how the resident's issues might be addressed.

Improper Reason: Keeping Others Awake

"Your mother is a screamer—her dementia causes her to moan and yell at night. She's preventing other residents from sleeping, which endangers their health. For the sake of other residents, she must be transferred."

Why the nursing home is wrong. Lack of sleep is not endangerment of health or safety. A resident generally doesn't endanger others' health unless she has a contagious condition that cannot be treated or quarantined. A better response on the part of the nursing home is to reassess the resident and identify new strategies to deal with her nighttime yelling.

Improper Reason: Striking Staff Members

"Your father waves his arms around whenever someone touches him. He struck a nurse aide yesterday in the arm. The nursing home could be financially liable if he were to cause an injury."

Why the nursing home is wrong. A resident generally doesn't endanger others' safety unless he attacks others physically and is strong and coordinated enough to do some real damage. Fear of financial liability is not a reason for eviction.

This guide recognizes that some residents behave in disruptive and disturbing ways. In most cases, such behavior is the result of dementia. The response should be care planning and treatment rather than eviction.

In this case, the staff might take special care to speak to the resident before touching him. Individuals with dementia can react aggressively when touched unexpectedly. The nursing home could identify an aide who works well with the resident and permanently assign the aide to work with him.

Improper Reason: Violation of Facility Policies

"You have been drinking beer, and drinking any alcoholic beverage is against facility policy. You must leave."

Why the nursing home is wrong. The resident has not endangered anyone's health or safety. Violation of facility policy is not one of the legitimate reasons for eviction.

Improper Reason: Resident Refuses Medical Treatment

"You have refused medical treatments that you do not like, and you do not cooperate with your dietary restrictions."

Why the nursing home is wrong. Like any other individual, a nursing home resident has a right to refuse medical treatment, as discussed in detail on page 143. As long as the refusal does not endanger others' health or safety, the resident's refusal of treatment does not justify eviction.

One exception to this rule is that a nursing home may be able to enforce a conscience-based policy requiring medical treatment if the nursing home had informed the resident of this policy before the resident was admitted. As a practical matter, this exception generally applies only to nursing homes affiliated with certain religious denominations that believe, as a matter of religious doctrine, that life-sustaining treatment always should be provided, even to terminally ill residents with limited or negligible prospects for recovery. See page 142 for additional discussion of this issue.

Improper Reason: Resident Does Not Need Nursing Home's Specialized Care

"This nursing home specializes in wound care, and you no longer need wound care."

Why the nursing home is wrong. The resident continues to need nursing home care. A resident's need for a stable living situation is more important than a nursing home's desire to specialize.

Do eviction laws apply to nursing home units in hospitals and to other nursing homes that generally provide short-term care?

Yes. The eviction laws apply to all nursing homes certified to accept payment from the Medicare and Medicaid programs, no matter the average length of a resident's stay in the nursing home. For example, a hospital's transitional care unit (which is certified as a nursing home) must follow the eviction laws outlined in this chapter.

Note that, in most cases, financial reasons prevent a resident from staying for an extended period in a hospital's nursing home unit. The rate charged by a hospital's nursing home unit is likely to be much higher than the rate charged by regular nursing homes. Neither residents nor Medicaid programs are willing to pay that rate when less expensive care in a regular nursing home is an option.

Does a denial of payment by the Medicare program or an HMO automatically justify a resident's eviction?

No. Such denials are not among the five legitimate reasons for eviction. In addition, a denial by the Medicare program or an HMO is not equivalent to nonpayment: such a denial does not prevent the nursing home from receiving payments from the resident, the Medicaid program, or another source.

Of course, if payment is not made from any source, the resident can be evicted for nonpayment.

What can be done if the Medicaid program refuses to pay for the care of a Medicaid-eligible resident and the nursing home seeks to evict the resident for nonpayment?

In a time of tight state budgets, Medicaid coverage of nursing home care is being squeezed from all directions. Because nursing home care is expensive, state Medicaid programs are often quick to terminate Medicaid coverage for a resident's nursing home care. Terminations are usually based on a finding that the resident no longer needs nursing home care; occasionally, terminations result from a mistake in the nursing home's request for reimbursement.

When a Medicaid program refuses to pay for a resident's care, nursing homes usually issue eviction notices based on nonpayment or on the grounds that care is no longer needed. In most cases, the resident or his representative should respond by immediately appealing both the proposed eviction and the Medicaid denial. These are two separate appeals—both are generally advisable.

The appeal of the eviction helps to protect the resident's place in the nursing home while the Medicaid appeal is pending. The resident will likely win the eviction appeal on the grounds that the nursing home served the eviction notice while the nursing home still was being paid.

Medicaid appeals are often successful. When the termination is based on the Medicaid program's argument that the resident does not

---

WORD TO THE WISE . . .

Point out mistakes. If the Medicaid termination occurred because the nursing home mishandled the Medicaid application or gave the resident inaccurate information about Medicaid, the nursing home's mistakes should be brought up in any eviction hearing. Nonpayment should not be grounds for eviction if the nonpayment was the nursing home's fault.

need nursing home care, the resident or his representative should be prepared to explain why the resident could not receive adequate care in an assisted living facility or at home. The resident's doctor can be very helpful. Ideally, the nursing home should assist the resident in his appeal with the Medicaid program—it is in the nursing home's interest that the resident's Medicaid coverage be resumed.

Can a nursing home evict a resident because she has become eligible for Medicaid?

Generally no, as long as the nursing home is certified for Medicaid. But rules vary from state to state.

In some states, Medicaid certification must apply to every bed in a nursing home (as discussed on p. 14). Other states allow a nursing home to certify only a portion of its beds.

In states that require complete Medicaid certification, a Medicaid-certified nursing home must accept Medicaid as payment whenever a private-pay resident spends her money down to Medicaid levels. The nursing home simply begins billing Medicaid for the resident's care; the conversion from private payment to Medicaid payment cannot be considered nonpayment.

In states that allow partial Medicaid certification, only designated rooms are certified for Medicaid reimbursement. When a private-pay resident spends her money down to Medicaid levels, she can stay in the nursing home only if a Medicaid room is available. Otherwise, she is at risk of being evicted due to nonpayment because the nursing home cannot bill Medicaid unless the resident is in a Medicaid-certified room.

Can a resident be evicted for nonpayment if he has become Medicaid-eligible but the nursing home has withdrawn from the Medicaid program?

No, not if the resident already had been admitted to the nursing home before the nursing home withdrew from Medicaid.

Q & A: MEDICAID CERTIFICATION

Q. I live in a state that allows a nursing home to certify only a portion of its rooms. Can I do anything to protect myself if I'm in a nursing home room that is not certified for Medicaid but my monthly nursing home bills will make me Medicaid-eligible within a few months?

A. Yes. As soon as possible, request in writing that the nursing home certify your room for Medicaid reimbursement. Federal law allows nursing homes to request certification of additional rooms. If the nursing home fails to certify your room and instead tries to evict you for nonpayment, you can point out in any eviction hearing that the nonpayment was caused by the nursing home's failure to get Medicaid certification for your room.

The size of the nursing home's Medicaid-certified area is under the nursing home's control. A nursing home can always choose to certify all of its rooms for Medicaid certification, even in those states that allow partial certification.

Federal law protects residents from having Medicaid certification pulled out from under them. It would be unfair if a resident chose a nursing home in part because the nursing home was Medicaid-certified and the nursing home could then deny Medicaid reimbursement by withdrawing from the Medicaid program.

Under the reform law, when a nursing home withdraws from the Medicaid program, the withdrawal does not affect any resident already in the nursing home at the time of the withdrawal. This protection applies whether the resident is Medicaid-eligible at the time of withdrawal or becomes eligible later.

SOME IMPROPER REASONS FOR EVICTION

- Time-consuming care needs
- Difficult behavior
- Keeping others awake
- Striking staff members
- Violation of facility policies
- Refusing medical treatment
- No need for nursing home's specialized care
- Nursing home is part of hospital complex
- Medicare or HMO reimbursement has ended
- Any other reason discussed on previous pages

Eviction Procedures

What notice of eviction must a nursing home give?

A nursing home must give adequate written notice of an eviction to the resident and to an immediate family member or legal representative. Generally, the notice must be given at least thirty days before the planned eviction, although under some circumstances the notice needs to be given only a "practicable" period of time before the planned eviction. In these cases, practicable notice should be long enough for the resident to obtain a hearing decision on an appeal before the planned eviction.

The notice must specify the reason for the eviction as well as the date of the eviction and the location to which the resident is to be moved. In addition, the notice must inform the resident and family that they can appeal the nursing home's decision to the appropriate state agency. Accordingly, the notice must list the telephone numbers and addresses for the state agency and the appropriate Long-Term Care Ombudsman program.

> ## WORD TO THE WISE . . .
>
> *Don't assume that the nursing home is right.* A resident and family should not assume that a nursing home's reasons are valid. As discussed, nursing homes often cite improper reasons for eviction.

Does a resident's doctor have to approve an eviction?

Yes, but only in two situations—when the resident's care needs allegedly cannot be met in a nursing home and when the resident no longer needs a nursing home. This requirement makes sense. If an eviction is supposedly for the resident's own good, the eviction at least should be supported by the resident's own doctor.

How can a resident appeal a nursing home's decision to evict her?

A resident or family member can appeal an eviction notice by contacting the state agency listed on the appeal form. Immediately after receiving a notice, the resident or family member should telephone the listed agency to request an appeal. In addition, the resident or family member should mail a dated appeal request to the state agency and keep a copy.

How should a resident or family member prepare for a hearing?

The resident or family member should focus on the five legitimate reasons for an eviction and prepare to show that none of those five reasons applies to the resident's situation. Specifically, the resident or family member should show that the nursing home's supposed reasons are not among the five legitimate reasons for an eviction or that the facts do not support any of the five legitimate reasons.

The resident or family member should obtain copies of relevant documents from the nursing home. Documents can be used to show, for example, that the nursing home failed to address the alleged problem through care planning or that it intends to transfer the resident to a nursing home that is not any better equipped to meet the resident's needs. A resident's right to copies of nursing home documents is discussed on pages 108–9.

Nursing home residents and their families may wish to be represented at the hearing by a knowledgeable attorney or other advocate. The resident or family may wish to bring witnesses, including family members, friends, and the resident's family doctor. A Long-

PARTIAL CHECKLIST OF DEFENSES

- The nursing home cannot prove one of the five legitimate reasons for eviction.
- The nursing home is responsible for the problem—for example, by failing to address the resident's dementia-related problems or, in a nonpayment case, by making mistakes in billing the Medicaid program.
- The nursing home alleges that the resident needs care that cannot be provided in a nursing home, but the resident's doctor has not documented the alleged need.
- The nursing home alleges that the resident needs care that cannot be provided in a nursing home, but this claim is false because the nursing home proposes to transfer the resident to another nursing home.
- The notice of the proposed eviction does not comply with the legal requirements (discussed earlier). For example, the notice does not specify the location to which the resident was to be sent, or fails to notify the resident of his appeal rights.
- The nursing home has not performed adequate discharge planning.

Term Care Ombudsman program representative, if knowledgeable about the resident's situation, may also be included (see pp. 172–73 for more about the ombudsman program).

A resident or family member should feel free to request and attend a hearing even if not represented by an attorney or other advocate. Residents and family can be successful in explaining why eviction is inappropriate.

How is an appeal conducted?

The state agency schedules the hearing. In most cases, the hearing is held at the nursing home. At that hearing, a hearing officer listens to the opinions of the resident, the resident's family members, the nursing home staff, and any other witnesses.

What types of arguments should a resident or family member make at a hearing?

The resident or family member should focus on the five legitimate reasons for eviction and show why none of those reasons apply. If appropriate, the resident or family member should point out how the nursing home's inadequacies may have caused the supposed problems. If, for example, the nursing home failed to address the resident's behavioral issues, the facility may bear significant responsibility for the resident's actions.

The resident or family member should point out any deficiencies in the nursing home's notice or procedure. A proposed eviction is frequently denied because the nursing home failed to follow the proper procedure.

Should the resident be at the hearing even if he is not competent mentally to testify?

Yes, or, at a minimum, the family member should arrange for the hearing officer to visit the resident in his room. Most residents present a sympathetic picture in person.

WORD TO THE WISE . . .

Be strong at the hearing. An eviction hearing can be intimidating, at least at first. Residents and family members are usually outnumbered at hearings. In a typical case concerning a resident's behavior, a nursing home is likely to have three to six employees testify about the resident's conduct.

Nursing homes' presentations at hearings tend to have an accusatory tone, suggesting that the resident has misbehaved and as a result deserves to be evicted. The resident or family members need to remind the hearing officer that nursing homes are designed to care for residents with dementia and other difficult conditions.

If possible, residents and family members should change the focus to mistakes that the nursing home may have made. The nursing home's mistakes are relevant legally, and pointing out the nursing home's mistakes can give the resident and family members confidence and momentum in their presentations to the hearing officer.

When does the hearing officer make a decision?

The hearing officer may rule at the conclusion of the hearing but will more likely issue a written decision later. Usually, the decision is issued within a week or two after the hearing, if not earlier.

What happens after the decision is issued?

If the resident wins, of course, she has the right to remain in the nursing home. If the resident loses but believes that the decision was wrong, she should immediately consult an attorney to consider appealing the decision.

WORD TO THE WISE . . .

Hearing officers can vary. Some hearing officers enforce the reform law stringently; others tend to give nursing homes the benefit of the doubt in virtually any situation. In the latter case, a resident who loses an appeal should consider appealing the hearing officer's ruling.

Must a nursing home help prepare a resident for transfer or discharge?

Yes. A nursing home must adequately prepare a resident for any transfer or discharge, whether voluntary or involuntary. Federal guidelines state that this preparation could include, among other actions, allowing a resident trial visits to his new home or ensuring that a resident does not lose his personal possessions.

Readmission after Absences from the Nursing Home: Bed-Hold Rules

Does a resident lose her nursing home bed by going to a hospital for a period of time?

It depends. Many states have bed-hold laws that require a nursing home to allow a resident to hold a nursing home bed during a hospital stay. The length of a required bed hold varies—an average required length is ten days.

A private-pay resident must pay for a bed hold himself. State Medicaid programs will generally pay for these bed holds for residents eligible for Medicaid reimbursement. The Medicare program does not pay for bed holds, although a nursing home resident whose care is reimbursed through Medicare may choose to pay for a bed hold himself.

The federal Nursing Home Reform Law requires that a nursing home notify a resident of the nursing home's bed-hold policy. Notice must be given at two times—when the resident first is admitted to the nursing home and whenever the resident is transferred from the nursing home to a hospital.

WORD TO THE WISE . . .

A resident's contract may give the right to a bed hold. A private-pay resident is arguably entitled to a bed hold of any length, even if state law requires only a short bed hold or doesn't mention bed holds at all. The resident has a contract with the nursing home: the nursing home provides a bed and services as long as the bill is paid. So if the resident continues to pay the bill, the resident should be able to hold the bed even if he is in the hospital for several weeks or longer. Of course, a bed hold of several weeks makes sense only if a resident is determined to hang onto his place in a particular nursing home and has enough money to justify spending it on a vacant nursing home bed.

Is there any additional protection for a Medicaid-eligible resident who is in a hospital beyond the state's required bed-hold period?
Yes. When a Medicaid-eligible resident is ready to leave the hospital, she is entitled to the nursing home's next available bed, even if the bed-hold period has long since expired.[1] A bed is not considered available if the roommate is a woman and the returning resident is a man or vice versa.

This rule is fair to the returning resident and the nursing home. To give the resident some stability, the nursing home is merely required to admit the resident to a vacant bed.

WORD TO THE WISE . . .

Ask promptly and consider whether to use Medicaid patient pay amount for bed hold. If the absence of a Medicaid-eligible resident has exceeded the bed-hold period, the resident should ask the nursing home for readmission to the next available bed as soon as he knows when he will be discharged from the hospital. It is unimportant whether the nursing home has a vacancy that day—the resident has a right to the next available bed, whenever it becomes available.

On rare occasions, readmission to the next available bed may not be adequate—for example, if the nursing home is unlikely to have any vacancies in the foreseeable future or if the resident just doesn't want to deal with the uncertainty of waiting for the next vacancy. In this case, a Medicaid-eligible resident may be able to pay for an extended bed hold by designating his monthly Medicaid patient pay amount to payment for the vacant nursing home bed. This plan will work only if the resident has a relatively high patient pay amount.

Assume, for example, that a resident owes $1,500 monthly as a Medicaid patient pay amount (also called a *share of cost*) and his nursing home bed costs $150 per day. After Medicaid pays for a limited bed hold—a week, for example—the resident could designate the $1,500 as payment for ten additional bed-hold days. Once the $1,500 deductible was met, the Medicaid program would pick up remaining health care expenses. (This plan would work only if the resident had not already paid the month's patient pay amount.)

This plan is one example of a general strategy in which a resident with a substantial patient pay amount may designate the patient pay amount for "extra" health care rather than for payment of regular nursing home charges. The advantage for the resident is that the Medicaid program will pay for nursing home charges once the patient pay amount is met. By designating the patient pay amount toward the extra health care—in this case, a vacant nursing home bed—the resident is able to receive the extra health care along with regular health care and nursing home services without paying more than the patient pay amount. More information about this general strategy is available on pages 52–53.

What can a resident do if a nursing home refuses to honor a bed hold or fails to comply with the legal obligation to readmit a Medicaid-eligible resident to the next available bed?

Despite the law, a nursing home sometimes refuses to readmit a resident after a hospital stay. The nursing home generally argues that it can no longer meet the resident's needs and thus is excused from the bed hold and readmission laws. In practice, this argument is almost always false—the nursing home can actually meet the resident's needs but sees an opportunity to rid itself of a resident whom it considers difficult or unprofitable.

If presented with this situation, the resident and family must act quickly. The hospital will likely want to discharge the resident in short order.

The resident and family should seek the advice of a knowledgeable attorney as soon as possible. The attorney may be able to get a court order to force the nursing home to readmit the resident.

Another option is for the resident or family member to make a complaint to the state inspection agency. (Contact information is in appendix C.) The resident or family member must emphasize to the inspection agency that immediate action is required. California and Oregon have administrative hearing procedures to handle a nursing home's refusal to readmit a resident from a hospital.

Q & A: BED HOLDS AND MEDICAID

Q. My mother is Medicaid-eligible. She was moved from her nursing home to a hospital when she had a heart attack. She is now stable and will be ready to go back to the nursing home in a few days. Is the nursing home required to readmit her?

A. Since your mother is Medicaid-eligible, the Medicaid program will likely pay to hold her nursing home bed. The maximum length of this bed hold varies from state to state.

If your mother's absence has exceeded the maximum bed-hold period, she is entitled to the next available Medicaid-certified bed. If your mother has a substantial Medicaid monthly patient pay amount, she may wish to designate her patient pay amount to pay for a bed hold beyond the bed hold paid for by the Medicaid program.

Transfers within a Nursing Home

Can a resident refuse a transfer from a Medicare-certified room to a room not certified for Medicare?

Yes. Under the Nursing Home Reform Law, a resident has the right to refuse a transfer from one room to another if the purpose of that transfer is to shift the resident from a Medicare room to a non-Medicare room. Usually when such a transfer is proposed, the resident is not entitled to Medicare reimbursement for his nursing home stay, but he could pay privately or arrange for Medicaid reimbursement, if eligible.

Nursing homes often claim that a Medicare-certified room must be occupied by a resident who currently is receiving Medicare reimbursement for his nursing home stay. This claim is false. In fact, a room's Medicare certification does not prevent it from being used by a resident paying privately or by a Medicaid-eligible

WORD TO THE WISE . . .

Act quickly to avoid being dumped at the hospital. Don't let a nursing home abandon a hospitalized resident. The nursing home is trying to evade the eviction procedures set by federal law. In the same way that an apartment landlord cannot change locks on an apartment when a tenant goes out of town for a weekend, a nursing home cannot discharge a resident against his will just because he was hospitalized for a few days. If a nursing home argues that a resident is, for example, a danger to others' safety, the nursing home should readmit the resident and then start eviction procedures.

When a nursing home appears resistant to readmission, it may seem easier for a resident and family to find a new nursing home where the resident is wanted than to do the advocacy work necessary to reclaim a bed in the original nursing home. However, keep in mind that a new nursing home may be no better—and might be worse—than the original nursing home. Also, the resident and family would likely prefer the familiar environment of the original nursing home. And if the resident and family take a stand and win, they may find themselves treated with greater attention and respect at the original nursing home.

resident, assuming that the bed is also certified for Medicaid reimbursement.

Can a resident contest a transfer from one room to another or the change of a roommate?

As discussed, a resident can refuse a room-to-room transfer if the purpose of the transfer is to move the resident out of a Medicare-certified room. A resident can also refuse a transfer if the purpose

WORD TO THE WISE . . .

Don't hesitate to refuse transfer. The law described here—allowing a resident to reject any Medicare-motivated transfer—was written to counterbalance reimbursement rules that give nursing homes a financial incentive to shuttle residents in and out of Medicare-certified rooms.

As discussed on pages 38–42, the Medicare program pays for a resident's nursing home care for only a limited period. Because Medicare pays a relatively high reimbursement rate, a nursing home has an incentive to move a resident out of a Medicare-certified room as soon as her eligibility for Medicare reimbursement has ended so that the nursing home can use the room for a resident eligible for Medicare reimbursement.

A resident should not be shy about asserting her right to remain in a Medicare-certified room if remaining in that particular room is important to her. In many instances, a nursing home assigns more-qualified staff to Medicare-certified rooms. A move away from a particular room may also be disorienting to the resident, or the original room may be preferable for some other reason.

If a nursing home complains that its Medicare-certified rooms could be filled by residents not eligible for Medicare reimbursement, the nursing home should be reminded that it can certify additional beds for Medicare reimbursement.

of the transfer is to move the resident to a Medicare-certified room, but in practice a resident rarely or never has reason to refuse a transfer for this reason.

Otherwise, the Nursing Home Reform Law requires only that a resident "receive notice before the room or roommate of the resident in the facility is changed." The resident generally has no right to refuse or appeal the transfer. In Indiana, a transfer within a nursing home is allowed only under limited circumstances.[2]

It may or may not be proper for a nursing home to transfer a resident who has just become Medicaid-eligible from one room to another. In a state that requires entire-facility certification as a condition for Medicaid reimbursement, such a move is improper, since all rooms are Medicaid-certified and the resident can access Medicaid reimbursement regardless of which room he is in. If a resident is nonetheless moved as a result of becoming Medicaid-eligible, the nursing home is evidently discriminating illegally on the basis of Medicaid eligibility.

In a state that allows a nursing home to certify only a portion of its rooms for Medicaid, a resident who becomes Medicaid-eligible may be required to move from one room to another in order to access Medicaid reimbursement. Residents in Medicaid-certified rooms should receive at least the same quality of care as that received by the nursing home's other residents.

Notes

1. The regulation requiring readmission to the next available bed is found at section 483.12(b)(3) of Title 42 of the Code of Federal Regulations.

2. Indiana law allows a transfer within a nursing home "only if the transfer is necessary for medical reasons as judged by the attending physician; or the transfer is necessary for the welfare of the resident or other persons." This regulation is found at section 16.2-3.1-12 of Title 410 of the Indiana Administrative Code.

9

How to Resolve Problems

- Introduction
- Organizing to Influence Care
- Resolving Problems

Introduction

This chapter suggests strategies for ensuring that a nursing home complies with the law and provides the care that nursing home residents deserve. The right strategy to use depends on the situation and, to a great extent, on the personality and preferences of the resident or family member. This chapter first reviews the rights of residents and their families to organize councils, and then it discusses methods to resolve nursing home problems.

Organizing to Influence Care

Do residents have the right to organize themselves?

Yes, residents have the right under the Nursing Home Reform Law to establish and maintain a resident council. If a resident council

---

WORD TO THE WISE . . .

You have a right to good care. Don't feel timid about requesting that the nursing home satisfy its legal obligations to provide good care. It's the nursing home that should be embarrassed if it has failed in its duty to provide high-quality care to you or your family member. The nursing home may claim that it is following standard operating procedures, but, as explained throughout this guide, a good number of these procedures are illegal.

Don't be discouraged if you initially make no progress in your discussions with nursing home staff and management. Be persistent. Once they understand that you will not give up, they may increasingly be inclined to make the changes that you want.

---

forms, the nursing home must provide the council with a private meeting space and designate a nursing home staff member as a contact person.

A nursing home must consider and respond to all complaints or recommendations made by a resident council.

WORD TO THE WISE . . .

Organizing can pay off. This guide recommends that residents put time and energy into organizing an effective resident council. Think big, but also recognize small victories. How powerful it would be if even five or ten residents got together to request a change in nursing home policy.

Resident councils can be powerful but are tremendously underutilized in practice. Many nursing homes do not have them. Even in those nursing homes with resident councils, the councils' agendas and activities are frequently set by the nursing home staff.

In part, resident councils are hindered by an inescapable fact—many nursing home residents have physical or mental limitations that prevent them from speaking up for themselves. But a bigger problem is that residents are uncomfortable challenging nursing home policies.

How can family members as a group influence the care provided by a nursing home?

Family members have the right to form a family council. The law on family councils is similar to the law on resident councils. A nursing home must provide a meeting space and a contact person and must consider and respond to all complaints and recommendations.

At their best, family councils are powerful organizations. A resident's family member can work within a family council to pressure a nursing home into making necessary improvements.

WORD TO THE WISE . . .

Again, organizing is key. Family councils, like resident councils, are often not as effective as they could be. This guide encourages family councils to think creatively about how the nursing home can be improved. Be prepared for some resistance from the nursing home, but also be prepared to explain how changes might make day-to-day life better for all concerned.

Resolving Problems

How can a resident or family member document a problem?

If a resident or family member believes that there is a problem with nursing home care, the resident may benefit by being seen by a different doctor or other health care professional. The resident has a right to receive such visits, as discussed on pages 97–99, assuming that the resident or resident's representative has consented.

Payment for this additional health care may be difficult for residents without much money. In some cases, the visit or examination will be covered by the Medicare or Medicaid programs. Also, a Medicaid-eligible resident with a monthly patient pay amount may be able to pay any uncovered charges by designating the patient pay amount toward those charges. This Medicaid strategy is discussed in detail on pages 52–53.

In discussing problems with nursing home staff and others, it is often helpful to use the relevant records from the resident's medical file at the nursing home. As discussed on pages 108–9, a resident or resident's representative has the right to review those records and receive copies.

It can also be helpful if a resident or family member can keep a written record of relevant events so that the resident or family member does not have to rely so heavily on memory. For example, a resident may record how frequently she is being turned, or a family member might keep a day-to-day log of the resident's appearance and condition.

How can a nursing home problem be resolved informally?

If a resident or family member has a problem with a nursing home, he should first talk to the nurse or nurse aide on duty. If the problem persists, the resident or family member should talk to a supervisor—the charge nurse—and then work up the chain of command to the nursing home's director of nursing or admin-

WORD TO THE WISE . . .

Develop relationships with staff members. Family members (and residents too) shouldn't overlook the value of being on good terms with nursing home staff. Chat with the nurses and nurse aides and, if it feels right, bring small gifts on special occasions. Everyday cordial behavior will make your complaints more credible, if a problem develops at some later time.

istrator. If necessary, the resident or family member should request a care plan meeting. Care plans are discussed on pages 112–14.

When discussing a problem, the resident or family member should listen carefully to the nursing home's position. Many problems can be resolved through discussion and negotiation if the resident, family member, and nursing home staff member are willing to listen to each other.

Whenever possible, the resident or family member should rely on legal requirements—for example, the laws explained in this guide. A nursing home cannot legally refuse to perform a service

IF I'M HAVING PROBLEMS, WHAT SHOULD I DO?

1. Talk to the nursing home staff.
2. Call the ombudsman program.
3. File a complaint with the state inspection agency.
4. Consult with an attorney.
5. Detailed instructions are provided in *20 Common Nursing Home Problems—and How to Resolve Them*, available from the National Senior Citizens Law Center at www.nsclc.org and 202-289-6976, ext. 201.

that the law requires. If a nursing home is not following the law, the resident or family member should not back down.

What organization will help a resident or family member discuss problems with a nursing home?

Sometimes a resident or family member will not make any progress by discussing a problem with nursing home staff. The resident or family member may then wish to call the local Long-Term Care Ombudsman program for assistance.

An ombudsman is someone who investigates reported complaints and helps to achieve settlements. The ombudsman program,

---

WORD TO THE WISE . . .

Allow an ombudsman program to identify a resident by name. As a practical matter, an ombudsman program in most cases cannot resolve a problem without revealing the name of the resident involved.

Residents and family members should not worry unduly about the nursing home retaliating against a resident in response to a complaint made by the resident or resident's family. Most states have laws prohibiting such retaliation.

More important, the real danger is not that a resident will be marked as a troublemaker but that the nursing home will identify a resident and the resident's family as customers who will put up with virtually anything. As mentioned, the squeaky wheel does generally get the grease in nursing homes. Residents and their families do themselves no favors by putting up with substandard care. Residents will benefit if they and their families thank the nursing home staff for good care but demand improvement whenever the quality of care falls short.

established by federal and state law, is completely independent from the nursing home.

Ombudsman program representatives are consumer advocates who attempt to ensure that nursing home residents have their problems heard and their rights protected. Ombudsman program representatives visit nursing homes to investigate possible concerns of residents. They also investigate problems in response to reported complaints.

A person reporting a problem to the ombudsman program can keep her name confidential, if desired. Similarly, the person reporting the problem may decide whether or not to participate in discussions between the ombudsman program and the nursing home.

Many ombudsman programs are staffed primarily by volunteers. In part because of the frequent reliance on volunteers, ombudsman programs differ greatly from each other in quality and capacity.

A state-by-state listing of ombudsman program contact information is provided in appendix B.

How can a resident or family member report a nursing home to the appropriate government agency?

If a resident or family member gets unsatisfactory results by talking with staff members, the resident or family member may wish to contact the state inspection agency.

A resident or family member can make a complaint (confidential or otherwise) concerning any nursing home. After investigating the complaint, the state agency may (1) force the nursing home to fix a problem, (2) force the nursing home to fix a problem and pay a fine or undergo some other penalty, or (3) find that the nursing home has broken no law.

Residents or family members requesting an investigation by the state inspection agency should submit complaints to the agency in writing to ensure that an inspector understands the problem. Any complaint should describe all the relevant information in a well-organized manner.

A state-by-state listing of state inspection agency contact information is provided in appendix C.

Can a resident or family member go to court to improve conditions in a nursing home?

Yes. A resident or family member may file a lawsuit against a nursing home to force the nursing home to comply with the law. For example, a personal injury action may be appropriate if a nursing home's action (or inaction) has caused serious physical or emotional harm.

In addition, if a resident or family member can show that a nursing home breaks the law on an ongoing basis, she could file a lawsuit against the nursing home's unfair practices. In such a lawsuit, the resident or family member could obtain a court order that would force the nursing home to change and improve its way of doing business.

A resident or family member considering a lawsuit should consult an attorney for additional details.

2006 State-Specific Medicaid Resource and Income Allowances; Average Monthly Private Pay Rates

State	Resident Resource Allowance	At-Home Spouse Resource Allowance (Minimum of $19,908; Maximum of $99,540)	Resident's Personal Needs Allowance	At-Home Spouse Income Allowance (Minimum of $1603.75 [changes 7/1/06]; Maximum of $2,489)	Average Monthly Private Pay Rate
Alabama	$2,000	$25,000	$30.00	$1,604	$4,000
Alaska	2,000	99,540	75.00	2,488.50	varies by region

State	Resident Resource Allowance	At-Home Spouse Resource Allowance	Resident's Personal Needs Allowance	At-Home Spouse Income Allowance	Average Monthly Private Pay Rate
Arizona	$2,000	$19,908	$90.45	$1,604	$4507.06 (Pinal, Pima, and Maricopa counties) 4189.44 (Rest of AZ)
Arkansas	2,000	19,908	40.00	1,604	3,604
California	2,000	99,540	35.00	2,489	5,031
Colorado	2,000	99,540	50.00	1,603.75	5,092
Connecticut	1,600	19,908	59.00	1,603.75	7,905
Delaware	2,000	25,000	44.00	1,604	4,905
DC	4,000	19,908	70.00	1,603.75	Actual facility cost
Florida	2,000	99,540	35.00	1,604	3,300
Georgia	2,000	99,540	30.00	2,488.50	4,167.33
Hawaii	2,000	99,540	30.00	2,488.50	7,314
Idaho	2,000	20,000	40.00	1,604	4,219
Illinois	2,000	99,540	30.00	2,489	Actual daily facility cost times 30
Indiana	1,500	19,908	52.00	1,605	3,898
Iowa	2,000	24,000	30.00	2,488.50	3,697.55
Kansas	2,000	19,908	30.00	1,604	3,000
Kentucky	2,000	20,000	40.00	1603.75	2,796
Louisiana	2,000	99,540	38.00	2,488.50	3,000

State	Resident Resource Allowance	At-Home Spouse Resource Allowance	Resident's Personal Needs Allowance	At-Home Spouse Income Allowance	Average Monthly Private Pay Rate
Maine	10,000	99,540	40.00	1,604	3,917
Maryland	2,500	19,908	60.00	1,604	4,300
Massachusetts	2,000	19,908	60.00	1,604	$232/ day*
Michigan	2,000	19,920	60.00	1,604	5,549
Minnesota	3,000	28,001	79.00	1,604	4,198
Mississippi	4,000	99,540	44.00	2,488.50	3,100
Missouri	1,000	19,908	30.00	1,604	2,758
Montana	2,000	19,908	40.00	1,604	4,292
Nebraska	4,000	19,908	50.00	1,652	Actual facility cost
Nevada	2,000	19,908	35.00	1,603.75	4,583
New Hampshire	2,500	19,908	56.00	1,604	6,467.90
New Jersey	2,000	19,908	35.00	1,604	6,525
New Mexico	2,000	31,290	54.00	1,604	4,541
New York	4,150	74,820	50.00	2,489	6,232 (Central) 9,842 (Long Island) 9,132 (New York City) 6,872 (North-eastern) 8,724

State	Resident Resource Allowance	At-Home Spouse Resource Allowance	Resident's Personal Needs Allowance	At-Home Spouse Income Allowance	Average Monthly Private Pay Rate
New York (continued)					(N. Metropolitan) 7,375 (Rochester) 6,540 (Western)
North Carolina	2,000	19,908	30.00	1,604	4,800
North Dakota	3,000	19,908	50.00	2,267	4,633
Ohio	1,500	19,908	40.00	1,604	4,806
Oklahoma	2,000	25,000	50.00	2,489	2,000
Oregon	2,000	19,908	30.00	1,604	5,050
Pennsylvania	2,400	19,908	40.00	1,604	6,062.35
Rhode Island	4,000	19,908	50.00	1,604	6,612
South Carolina	2,000	66,480	30.00	2,416	4,234
South Dakota	2,000	20,000	60.00	1,603.75	4,026.09
Tennessee	2,000	19,908	40.00	1,604	7,905
Texas	2,000	19,908	45.00	2,488.50	117.08/ day
Utah	2,000	19,908	45.00	1,603.75	3,618
Vermont	2,000	99,540	47.66	1,657	5,921
Virginia	2,000	19,908	30.00	1,603.75	5,403 Northern VA 4,060 Rest of VA

State	Resident Resource Allowance	At-Home Spouse Resource Allowance	Resident's Personal Needs Allowance	At-Home Spouse Income Allowance	Average Monthly Private Pay Rate
Washington	2,000	41,943	51.62	1,604	181/day
West Virginia	2,000	19,908	50.00	1,604	3,380
Wisconsin	2,000	50,000	45.00	2,488.50	5,096
Wyoming	2,000	99,540	50.00	2,488.50	4,686

Notes: These figures are current as of 1/31/06. States may change these figures throughout the year, so consumers and advocates should verify current levels with the local Medicaid office before relying on them for Medicaid long-term care eligibility calculations. Figure marked with an asterisk was in the process of changing at the time this publication went to press.

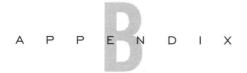

State Long-Term Care Ombudsman Programs

State	Address	Phone
Alabama	RSA Plaza #470 770 Washington Avenue Montgomery, AL 36130	334-242-5743
Alaska	550 West 7th Avenue, Suite 1830 Anchorage, AK 99501	907-334-4480
Arizona	1789 West Jefferson-950A Phoenix, AZ 85007	602-542-6454
Arkansas	P.O. Box 1437, Slot S530 Little Rock, AR 72203-1437	501-682-8952
California	1330 National Drive, Suite 200 Sacramento, CA 95834	916-419-7510
Colorado	455 Sherman Street, Suite 130 Denver, CO 80203	800-288-1376
Connecticut	25 Sigourney Street, 12th Floor Hartford, CT 06106-5033	860-424-5200

State	Address	Phone
Delaware	1901 North Dupont Highway Main Admin Bldg Annex New Castle, DE 19720	302-255-9390
DC	601 E Street, NW, A4-315 Washington, DC 20049	202-434-2140
Florida	4040 Esplanade Way Tallahassee, FL 32399	888-831-0404
Georgia	2 Peachtree Street, NW, 9th Floor Atlanta, GA 30303-3142	888-454-5826
Hawaii	250 South Hotel Street, Suite 406 Honolulu, HI 96813-2831	808-586-0100
Idaho	P.O. Box 83720 3380 American Terrace, Suite 120 Boise, ID 83720-0007	208-334-3833
Illinois	421 East Capitol Avenue, Suite 100 Springfield, IL 62701-1789	217-785-3143
Indiana	402 West Washington Street, Room W454 P.O. Box 7083, MS21 Indianapolis, IN 46207-7083	800-545-7763
Iowa	510 East 12th Street Jessie M. Parker Bldg, Suite 2 Des Moines IA 50319	515-725-3327
Kansas	900 SW Jackson Street, Suite 1041 Topeka, KS 66612	877-662-8362
Kentucky	275 East Main Street, 1E-B Frankfort, KY 40621	502-564-5497
Louisiana	412 North 4th Street, 3rd Floor P.O. Box 61 Baton Rouge, LA 70821	225-342-6872
Maine	1 Weston Court P.O. Box128 Augusta, ME 04332	207-621-1079
Maryland	301 West Preston Street, Room 1007 Baltimore, MD 21201	410-767-1100

State	Address	Phone
Massachusetts	1 Ashburton Place, 5th Floor Boston, MA 02108-1518	617-727-7750
Michigan	7109 West Saginaw P.O. Box 30676 Lansing, MI 48909	517-335-0148
Minnesota	P.O. Box 64971 St. Paul, MN 55164-0971	651-431-2555
Mississippi	750 North State Street Jackson, MS 39202	601-359-4927
Missouri	P.O. Box 570 Jefferson City, MO 65102	800-309-3282
Montana	P.O. Box 4210 111 North Sanders Helena, MT 59604-4210	406-444-7785
Nebraska	P.O. Box 95044 Lincoln, NE 68509-5044	402-471-2307
Nevada	445 Apple Street, Suite 104 Reno, NV 89502	775-688-2964
New Hampshire	129 Pleasant Street Concord, NH 03301-3857	603-271-4704
New Jersey	P.O. Box 807 Trenton, NJ 08625-0807	609-943-4026
New Mexico	1015 Tijeras Avenue, NW, Suite 200 Albuquerque, NM 87102	505-222-4500
New York	2 Empire State Plaza Agency Building #2 Albany, NY 12223	518-474-7329
North Carolina	2101 Mail Service Center Raleigh, NC 27699-2101	919-733-8395
North Dakota	600 East Boulevard Avenue, Dept. 325 Bismarck, ND 58505	800-451-8693
Ohio	50 West Broad Street, 9th Floor Columbus, OH 43215-3363	614-644-7922

State	Address	Phone
Oklahoma	2401 N.W. 23rd Street, Suite 40 Oklahoma City, OK 73107	405-521-6734
Oregon	3855 Wolverine NE, Suite 6 Salem, OR 97305-1251	503-378-6533
Pennsylvania	555 Walnut Street, 5th Floor P.O. Box 1089 Harrisburg, PA 17101	717-783-1550
Rhode Island	422 Post Road, Suite 204 Warwick, RI 02888	401-785-3340
South Carolina	1301 Gervais Street, Suite 200 Columbia, SC 29201	803-734-9900
South Dakota	700 Governors Drive Pierre, SD 57501-2291	605-773-3656
Tennessee	500 Deaderick Street, Suite 825 Nashville, TN 37243	615-741-2056
Texas	701 West 51st Street P.O. Box 149030, Mail Code 250 Austin, TX 78714-9030	512-438-4356
Utah	120 North, 200 West, Room 325 Salt Lake City, UT 84103	801-538-3910
Vermont	264 North Winooski Avenue P.O. Box 1367 Burlington, VT 05402	802-863-5620
Virginia	24 East Cary Street, Suite 100 Richmond, VA 23219	804-565-1600
Washington	1200 South 336th Street P.O. Box 23699 Federal Way, WA 98093	800-422-1384
West Virginia	1900 Kanawha Boulevard East Bldg #10 Charleston, WV 25305-0160	304-558-3317
Wisconsin	1402 Pankratz Street Madison, WI 53704-4001	800-815-0015
Wyoming	756 Gilchrist P.O. Box 94 Wheatland, WY 82201	307-322-5553

State Inspection Agencies

State	Address	Phone
Alabama	Department of Public Health 201 Monroe Street, RSA Tower Montgomery, AL 36104	334-206-5111
Alaska	Health Facilities Licensing & Certification 350 Main Street PO Box 110601 Juneau, AL 99811-0601	907-334-2483
Arizona	Department of Health Services 150 North 18th Avenue Phoenix, AZ 85007	602-364-2690
Arkansas	Department of Health Services 4815 West Markham Little Rock, AR 72205	501-682-8430
California	Department of Health Services Licensing and Certification MS 3000 P.O. Box 997413 Sacramento, CA 95899	916-552-8700

State	Address	Phone
Colorado	Department of Public Health & Environment 4300 Cherry Creek Drive, South Denver, CO 80246-1530	303-692-2800
Connecticut	Department of Health Services 410 Capitol Avenue, MS#12HSR Hartford, CT 06134-0308	860-509-7400
Delaware	Health and Social Services of Delaware—Division of Long Term Care and Resident Protection 3 Mill Road, Ste. 308 Wilmington, DE 19806	302-577-6661
District of Columbia	Department of Consumer & Regulatory Affairs 941 North Capitol Street, NE Washington, DC 20002	202-727-7190
Florida	Agency for Health Care Administration 2727 Mahan Drive Tallahassee, FL 32308	888-491-3456
Georgia	Department of Human Resources—Office of Regulatory Resources 2 Peachtree Street, NW #32-415 Atlanta, GA 30303-3167	404-657-9639
Hawaii	State Department of Health 1250 Punchbowl St. Honolulu, Hawaii 96813	808-692-7420
Idaho	Department of Health & Welfare 450 West State Street, 3rd Floor Boise, ID 83720-0036	208-334-6626
Illinois	Department of Public Health 535 West Jefferson Street Springfield, IL 62761	217-782-0321

State	Address	Phone
Indiana	State Department of Health— Long Term Care Division 2 North Meridian Street Indianapolis, IN 46204	317-233-7442
Iowa	Department of Inspections & Appeals Lucas State Office Building 321 East 12th Street Des Moines, Iowa 50319-0083	515-281-4115
Kansas	Department on Aging New England Building 503 S. Kansas Ave. Topeka, KS 66603-3404	785-296-4986
Kentucky	Office of Inspector General of Kentucky 275 East Main Street Frankfort, KY 40621	502-564-7963
Louisiana	Department of Health & Hospitals Health Standards Section 1201 Capitol Access Road P.O. Box 629 Baton Rouge, LA 70821	225-342-0148
Maine	Department of Human Services Division of Licensing and Certification 442 Civic Center Drive Augusta, ME 04333	207-287-9300
Maryland	Department of Health & Mental Hygiene Spring Grove Center 55 Wade Ave Catonville, MD 21228	410-402-8201
Massachusetts	Department of Public Health 250 Washington Street Boston, MA 02108-4619	617-753-8000

State	Address	Phone
Michigan	Department of Community Health Capitol View Building 201 Townsend Street Lansing, MI 48933	517-373-3740
Minnesota	Office of Health Facility Complaints P.O. Box 64970 St. Paul, MN 55164-0970	651-215-8702
Mississippi	State Department of Health 570 East Woodrow Wilson Drive Jackson, MS 39216	601-576-7300
Missouri	Elder Abuse and Neglect Hotline Division of Senior and Disability Services Missouri Department of Health and Senior Services PO Box 570 Jefferson City, MO 65102-0570	573-751-4842
Montana	Department of Public Health & Human Services Quality Assurance Division- Licensure Bureau 2401 Colonial Drive P.O. Box 202953 Helena, MT 59620-2953	406-444-2099
Nebraska	Department of Health and Human Services Regulation and Licensure Credentialing Division PO Box 94986 Lincoln, NE 68509	402-471-3324
Nevada	Department of Health & Human Services 505 East King Street, Room 600 Carson City, NV 89701-3708	775-687-4475

State	Address	Phone
New Hampshire	Bureau of Health Facilities Administration 129 Pleasant St. Concord, NH 03301-3857	603-271-4592
New Jersey	Department of Health & Senior Services P.O. Box 360 Trenton, NJ 08625-0360	609-633-8991
New Mexico	Department of Health of New Mexico—Bureau of Health Facility Licensing and Certification 1190 S. St. Francis Dr. Santa Fe, NM 87502	505-476-9025
New York	New York State Department of Health Corning Tower Empire State Plaza Albany, NY 12237	518-408-1162
North Carolina	Division of Facility Services DFS Webmaster 2701 Mail Service Center Raleigh, NC 27699-2701	919-855-4050
North Dakota	Department of Health 600 E. Boulevard Ave. Bismarck, ND 58505-0200	701-328-2352
Ohio	Department of Health Bureau of Long Term Care of Ohio—Quality Assurance 246 North High Street Columbus, OH 43215	614-752-9524
Oklahoma	State Department of Health 1000 NE 10TH Street Oklahoma City, OK 73117	405-271-6868

State	Address	Phone
Oregon	Department of Human Services Seniors and People with Disabilities 500 Summer St. NE Salem, OR 97301	503-945-5832
Pennsylvania	Department of Health Health and Welfare Building 7th & Forster Streets Harrisburg, PA 17120	717-787-1816
Rhode Island	Department of Health 3 Capitol Hill Providence, RI 02908	401-222-2566
South Carolina	Department of Health & Human Services Bureau of Certification P. O. Box 8206 Columbia, SC 29202-8206	803-545-4205
South Dakota	Department of Health Office of Licensure & Certification 615 E. 4th St. Pierre, SD 57501	605-773-3356
Tennessee	Department of Health 425 Fifth Avenue, North Cordell Hull Building, 3rd Floor Nashville, TN 37247	615-741-7221
Texas	Department of Aging and Disability Services 701 W. 51st St. Austin, TX 78751	512-438-2633
Utah	Department of Health Medicare/Medicaid Program Certification/Resident Assessment 4th Floor Cannon Health Building Box 141000 Salt Lake City, UT 84114-1000	801-538-6158

State	Address	Phone
Vermont	Agency of Human Services Department of Disabilities, Aging & Independent Living 103 South Main St. Waterbury, VT 05671	802-241-2345
Virginia	Department of Health Center for Quality Health Care Services and Consumer Protection P.O. Box 2448 Richmond, Virginia 23218-2448 109 Governor Street Richmond, Virginia 23219	804-367-2100
Washington	Department of Social & Health Services Aging & Disability Services Administration P.O. Box 45600 Olympia, WA 98504-5600	360-725-2300
West Virginia	Department of Health & Human Resources Office of Health Facility Licensure and Certification Capital and Washington Streets 1 Davis Square, Suite 101 Charleston, WV 25301-1799	304-558-0050
Wisconsin	Department of Health and Family Services Division of Supportive Living- Bureau of Quality Assurance 1 W. Wilson Street Madison, WI 53702	608-266-8481
Wyoming	Department of Health Office of Health Quality of Wyoming 401 Hathaway Building Cheyenne, WY 82002	307-777-7123

Index